Janetta M. Bauer Personal Property

Current Therapy of Communication Disorders

LANGUAGE HANDICAPS IN ADULTS

Current Therapy of Communication Disorders

LANGUAGE HANDICAPS IN ADULTS

edited by
William H. Perkins, Ph.D.
University of Southern California

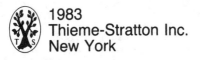

1983
Thieme-Stratton Inc.
New York

Georg Thieme Verlag
Stuttgart • New York

Acknowledgment

My unbounded gratitude to John Rosenbek for guidance in selection of topics for this volume is matched only by my gratitude for his assistance in obtaining authors for those topics.

Publisher: Thieme-Stratton Inc.
381 Park Avenue South
New York, New York 10016

Cover typography by M. Losaw

Printed in the United States of America

CURRENT THERAPY OF COMMUNICATION
DISORDERS
Language Handicaps in Adults
edited by William H. Perkins

TMP ISBN 0-86577-406-4 (pbk)

CONTENTS

CONTRIBUTING AUTHORS

Brenda L. Adamovich, Ph.D.
Braintree Hospital, Braintree, MA

Michael Collins, Ph.D.
Veterans Administration Hospital, Madison, WI

Lee Ann C. Golper, M.S.
Veterans Administration Medical Center, Portland, OR

Nancy Helm-Estabrooks, D.Sc.
Veterans Administration Medical Center, Boston, MA

Jennifer A. Henderson, M.S.
Braintree Hospital, Braintree, MA

Jennifer Horner, Ph.D.
Duke University Medical Center, Durham, NC

Michael G. Johnson, M.A., C.C.C.
Private practice, Minneapolis, MN

Judith L. Kennedy, M.S.
University of Rochester Medical Center, Rochester, NY

Iris Tanney Kraemer, M.A.
Veterans Administration Medical Center, Gainesville, FL

Leonard LaPointe, Ph.D.
Veterans Administration Medical Center, Gainesville, FL

Craig W. Linebaugh, Ph.D.
The George Washington University, Washington, D.C.

Penelope Starratt Myers, M.A., C.C.C.
The George Washington University, Washington, D.C.

Joan C. Payne-Johnson, Ph.D.
Howard University, Washington, D.C.

Marie T. Rau, M.S.
Veterans Administration Medical Center,
Portland, OR

Nina N. Simmons, M.S.
Louisiana Rehabilitation Institute, New Orleans, LA

Kathryn M. Yorkston, Ph.D.
Department of Rehabilitative Medicine, University of
Washington, WA

Wanda G. Webb, Ph.D.
Vanderbilt University, Nashville, TN

FOREWORD TO THE SERIES

Roughly a billion dollars is invested annually in clinical service of speech, language, and hearing disorders. Were this service provided to only one person, our best effort would be mandatory. The magnitude of the investment merely heightens the importance of our clinical responsibility.

The volumes in this series are an effort to help meet this responsibility. They are intended for the practicing clinician who needs a convenient reference for therapy of any problem of speech, language, or hearing. Each volume contains as many chapters as were required to present all of the forms of therapy which are currently differentiated for disorders of language, articulation, voice, fluency, and hearing in children and adults. One could call this a distinctive feature approach in the sense that therapy of any disorder that is distinguished from therapy of another disorder by at least one feature of treatment warranted a separate chapter.

To avoid repeating general procedures for learning new responses, transferring them to daily life, and making them permanent, they are presented in the volume, *General Principles of Therapy*. Each general technique is described from the standpoint of whatever theory of learning it is mainly derived. For example, response shaping is presented as an operant procedure, modeling as a procedure of cognitive learning theory. These procedures are not described systematically in the other volume. Instead, each chapter in these volumes is a free standing, terse, procedural account of a specific therapy as practiced by the author for a specific type of disorder.

The focus of this text is exclusively on treatment. Matters of assessment, diagnosis, and rationale are included only to the extent that they are needed to clarify characteristics of the person for whom the therapy is intended, and the reasons for it. Credibility of the therapy is embedded in credibility of the authors, who were selected on the best advice I could obtain. Asking them to describe what they do was tantamount to asking them to evaluate our treatment-research literature. Because they must make the most responsible judgment they can for each person they serve, their treatment recognizes the research which has therapy value and goes beyond science to include the intangible verities of clinical practice as an art.

William H. Perkins

PREFACE

I discovered quickly, when organizing this volume, what experts in aphasia have known all along—that classifying language handicaps of adults, aphasia in particular, is a hazardous business. Obviously, I had to select among alternatives. My choices of chapter topics were determined by posing this question to the wisest counsel I could find, "What are the types of language handicaps in adults that should be treated differently from each other?"

With these distinctions made, I then sought, with assistance, authors whose clinical experience strongly qualified them to address the particular features of treatment required for each type of problem. What emerged are the methods of therapy of astute clinical artist-scientists that are reported in this volume.

William H. Perkins

LANGUAGE HANDICAPS IN ADULTS

CHAPTER ONE

TREATMENT OF BROCA'S APHASIA

Method of Jennifer Horner

The treatment described is for the phonologic-syntactic expressive deficit in Broca's aphasia. Severity, chronicity, degree of residual language in other modalities, and memory/learning potential are significant prognostic considerations for response to treatment. Clinical techniques involve restitution of function (facilitation and prevention) and substitution of function (reorganization and compensation). The clinician's awareness of how the minor hemisphere may mediate language recovery may be critical to the success of clinical intervention.

THE CLINICAL PROBLEM

The expressive language of Broca's aphasia is nonfluent and agrammatic. I use the term "nonfluent" to refer to the phonologic-prosodic deficit. This deficit profile typically includes: (1) reduced rate, (2) reduced phrase length, (3) excessive initial and interstitial pause, and (4) aberrations in syllabic, phrasal, and sentence prosody (stress, pause, duration, and tone). I use the term "agrammatic" to refer to (1) absence or erroneous usage of inflectional morphemes and (2) absence or erroneous use of functors, usually occurring in the context of simplified or stereotyped sentence frames. With few exceptions, the Broca's aphasic patient also presents phonemically disordered speech characterized by sound selection errors and/or phonetic distortions in the context of initiation and sequencing difficulty, and abnormal prosody.

UNDERLYING ASSUMPTIONS

First, I adhere to the view that participation of the minor hemisphere is vital to the recovery of communication functions, particularly in the moderately or severely aphasic individual. While this is most

3

apparent in the chronic phase, I attempt to stimulate minor hemisphere participation in both the acute and chronic stages of recovery. Second, while syntactic comprehension deficits typically parallel syntactic expressive deficits, I believe that the social-pragmatic-functional impact of Broca's aphasia lies in the expressive realm, and this is where I begin therapy. I find that comprehension functions can be effectively treated indirectly in most cases by careful manipulation of stimulus inputs. My stimulus selection is guided not only by syntactic constraints, but also by immediate memory and lexical-semantic limitations. Comprehension can also be enhanced by inclusion of visual-nonphonetic stimuli, which stimulate minor hemisphere participation. Third, I assume that the expressive language function in all but the very mildly aphasic individual is fundamentally "altered," i.e., different from normal. In my experience, "normalization" of expressive functions is rarely a practicable goal. Instead, I attempt to help the aphasic patient to attain a level of speech that is socially acceptable and pragmatically flexible. For this reason, I give priority to clinical goals in the following order: (1) intelligibility, (2) pragmatic variety, and (3) length and complexity of sentences.

INITIAL OBSERVATIONS

During the initial interview, I observe the repertoire of spontaneous behaviors, both verbal and nonverbal, and I note potentially maladaptive behaviors. Regarding vocalization, absence of voice or vocal initiation difficulty often suggests a concomitant phonatory apraxia and may signal phonologic-prosodic aberrations in later stages of therapy. I note the variety and appropriateness of intonational variations, and the context in which they occur. I observe the repertoire of speech sounds (normal or reduced) and the variability of phonemic accuracy. I note the correlation of phonologic paraphasias with rate of speech, phrase length, and prosody. I observe the variety of grammatical forms. I also observe the patient's spontaneous use of elaborative gestures.

Potentially maladaptive behaviors are usually fairly obvious. These include: response impulsivity, struggle and frustration, overemphasis of vocalization and articulatory postures, equalization of stress in propositional utterances, as well as overuse and repetition of readily available forms in compensation for linguistic retrieval deficits.

In terms of receptive communicative behaviors, I observe the patient's attentiveness to extra-linguistic parameters of communication such as facial expression, visual-situational cues, elaborative gestures, and recognition of basic sentence types, i.e., recognition of social speech versus yes/no questions versus "wh" questions. I estimate overall communicative adequacy in terms of the overall amount of information conveyed, and the degree of independence assumed by the patient in the communicative exchange.

EXPRESSIVE LANGUAGE INVENTORY

I begin a language remediation program by obtaining a standardized baseline measure of auditory-verbal, visual-constructive, and reasoning abilities. I supplement standardized tests, as necessary, with comparative measures of spontaneous speech versus spontaneous writing, repetition, and oral reading.

I elicit spontaneous speech through conversation and presentation of pictures to be described. I then analyze fluency and grammar. I obtain a composite fluency measure as follows: "Language fluency" is estimated from measures of the length of grammatical phrases, and the intrusion of vocalized hesitations interpreted to be reflections of word-retrieval difficulty. "Speech fluency" is marked by prosodic boundaries and intra- or interstitial pause, and is measured in terms of average phrase length, maximum phrase length, and overall articulatory agility. I consider overall rate (words per minute) to be a general index of speech and language productivity and efficiency.

A grammatical analysis includes observations of simplified and/ or stereotyped sentence forms, the distribution and variety of contentives versus functors, and the omission and/or substitution of syntactic morphemes (inflectional morphemes and functors).

In order to identify the pervasiveness of the nonfluent-agrammatic deficit and to identify potentially facilitative modalities, I compare spontaneous speech with oral reading, repetition, and spontaneous writing in terms of phrase length, phoneme/grapheme accuracy, and syntactic integrity. I include tasks of limb praxis and constructional praxis (drawing and copying) to rule out modality-specific deficits that may confound expressive treatments.

RESTITUTION AND SUBSTITUTION THEORIES OF RECOVERY: CLINICAL APPLICATION

In the management of Broca's aphasia, I assume that two processes of recovery are active: a restitution process and a substitution process. The restitution of function theory accounts for the quantitative physiologic improvement of neural processes in the acute ("spontaneous recovery") phase. The substitution of function theory assumes that improvement results from reorganization within and across functional systems. Our role as clinicians in the acute phase is to maximize expressive behaviors through stimulation within each modality. This multimodality treatment may include: (1) copying, (2) serial writing (numbers and alphabet), (3) production of speech at the patient's level of breakdown (via imitation, sentence completion, and sentence formulation tasks), and (4) vocabulary enrichment drills (via written and spoken naming tasks and silent reading tasks). The goal of restitution treatments is to strengthen, reinstate, and enhance residual language while minimizing maladaptive behavior. Selected tasks engage intrahemispheric (auditory-verbal) processing. I employ the task continuum concept to organize treatment materials, and behavior modification methodology to elicit desired linguistic behaviors.

In contrast to restitution of function processes, substitution of function may occur during and beyond the acute phase of recovery. Under the auspices of this model, I believe that the role of the clinician is to provide strategies by which the patient can substitute qualitatively reorganized behavior for fundamentally altered language behavior. Reorganization strategies involve the combination of functional cortical systems in new and unprecedented ways to help the patient compensate for and circumvent language systems that are no longer viable. Reorganization strategies may involve either intra- or interhemispheric functional systems.

Minor Hemisphere Mediation

I use minor hemisphere mediation strategies in the treatment of moderately and severely impaired Broca's aphasic individuals. Three assumptions of this model are: (1) under appropriate stimulus conditions, the minor hemisphere can be tapped to mediate language recovery, (2) restoration of prosody (primarily a minor hemisphere ability) is necessary to phonologic-syntactic reorganization, and (3) the potential for phonologic-syntactic recovery is enhanced through systematic pairing of speech with visual-spatial-holistic stimuli, which engage minor hemisphere perceptual-cognitive processes.

While phonologic-syntactic processing is a dominant hemisphere function, visual-spatial-holistic processing is a minor hemisphere function in most individuals. Briefly, minor hemisphere perceptual-cognitive abilities available to the patient with isolated dominant hemisphere damage include: holistic perception of objects and faces; copying and drawing; musical-prosodic faculties; and emotional behavior, including recognition of affective speech and emotional gesturing. Selective attention and "intention" to respond are also minor hemisphere functions.

The term visual-spatial implies that visual receptive skills are superior to auditory, and that stimuli as they are organized in space are more readily processed than stimuli organized in time. The term holistic refers to events that occur as a whole, i.e., events that cannot readily be divided into discrete parts. Facial expressions, arm and hand gestures (including emotional and symbolic gestures), melodic patterns, objects, pictures, novel pictorial symbols, and some highly imageable and familiar printed words lend themselves to visual-spatial-holistic processing. In addition to being visual-spatial-holistic, these stimuli are distinguished from auditory-verbal stimuli because they are nonphonetic and ideographic.

It is from this armamentarium that I select treatment stimuli for the Broca's aphasic patient. I then systematically pair them with impaired phonologic-syntactic behaviors. Some factors that may influence the usefulness of visual-spatial-holistic strategies as reorganizers are: (1) premorbid cognitive style, (2) motivation to use a "reorganized" communication system, and (3) learning ability.

LINGUISTIC AND VISUAL-SPATIAL-HOLISTIC TREATMENT CONSIDERATIONS

The goal of treatment of the Broca's aphasic individual is production of basic sentence types that are phonologically and syntactically acceptable, in addition to being affective, informative, and pragmatically flexible. Planning an expressive remediation program for the nonfluent-agrammatic patient involves three overlapping factors: (1) prosodic contour, (2) phonologic form, and (3) syntactic form. Both linguistic considerations and visual-spatial-holistic considerations should ideally be integrated in treatment. I attempt to include hierarchical facilitation techniques in the general framework of a reorganization model as described in Table 1.

In all steps of a reorganization treatment, I control the linguistic complexity of utterances. I use task continua to identify the patient's performance ceiling. At this point, I work with homogeneous sets of stimuli below the patient's performance ceiling to enhance learning of the salient reorganizing strategy.

Linguistic Considerations

Prosodic contour. Stimuli are organized according to stress patterns. At the syllable and word level, I drill control of duration and

TABLE 1. Considerations for Auditory-Verbal Facilitation and Reorganization of Broca's Aphasia

Linguistic Considerations	*Visual-Spatial-Holistic Considerations*
Prosodic Contour	
Minimal Unit: Syllable Control linguistic stress pattern in syllables, words, and phrases	Minimal Unit: Syllable Associate facial expression with changes in stress, duration, and tone Associate holistic movements with changes in stress, duration, and tone
Phonologic Form	
Minimal Unit: Word (Holophrase) First treat holophrastic utterances Gradually increase utterance length Control form class Control phonetic complexity	Minimal Unit: Word (Ideogram) Pair speech with representational and symbolic gestures Pair speech with imageable printed words (teach whole word reading) Pair speech with novel pictorial symbols
Syntactic Form	
Minimal Unit: Phrase Treat basic sentence types Treat N, V, and ADJ equally Avoid syntactic redundancy Treat concatenation before embedded and reversible sentences Treat copying and writing simultaneously with verbal expression	Minimal Unit: Phrase Stabilize phonologic-prosodic features using frequently used and functional phrases Pair syntactic speech with sequences of symbolic gestures, imageable printed words, or novel pictorial symbols Use visual enhancement techniques (diacritical marks, tree diagrams) to aid memory and organization

tone. I begin with initial position stress and move the primary stress gradually from initial, to medial, to final position. The liberal and judicious use of pause is vital to establishing and maintaining prosodic patterns.

Phonologic form. I first establish a functional repertoire of holophrastic utterances, including expletives and contentives, because these are most readily available to the Broca's patient. I later add select functors such as "wh" words, nominal pronouns, and negatives. I consistently select words that are familiar, useful, and "pronounceable" in terms of phonetic complexity and visualization. The syllable is the minimal unit of phonologic retraining; I increase the length of utterances in small increments, typically to a ceiling of 6 to 8 syllables (3 to 5 words).

Syntactic form. In phonologic and syntactic retraining, I think the maximal length of utterances should not exceed the maximum phrase length observed in spontaneous speech, which is often comparable to the patient's auditory-verbal memory span. I am cautious not to sacrifice phonologic-prosodic gains for syntactic "normalcy." I organize homogeneous sets of syntactic materials according to several dimensions of sentence form: sentence type, form class, redundancy, and complexity.

I begin therapy with basic sentence types: declarative (N + V [+ O]) and imperative, in the present tense. I avoid overuse of nouns in treatment stimuli; instead, I treat nouns, verbs, and adjectives equally, when possible, to help the Broca's patient minimize the tendency to rely on nominal forms. I introduce adjectives in the sentence frame ([N or PRO] + is + ADJ). I introduce tense distinctions to verb forms as early in the treatment as possible, in this order: present progressive, regular past, and future.

I am careful to avoid "redundant" morphosyntactic forms in early stages of therapy. We know from the literature and from experience that Broca's patients omit unstressed inflections and functors that are not "informative," especially when word order and stress are sufficient to convey information about actor, action, agent, tense, possession, location, etc. I establish goals regarding morphosyntactic retraining based on what I think the individual's syntactic processing mechanism can effectively master. Some patients may effectively use rote memorization of frequently used structures, others may be able to learn morphosyntactic rules, and others may be unable to relearn morphosyntactic patterns. In all cases, I observe the clinical priorities stated earlier: intelligibility, first, and length and complexity of syntax, last.

On the other hand, I avoid teaching or reinforcing agrammatic speech patterns whenever possible. I use a technique I call "tagging," and I observe "syntactic preferences." "Tagging" refers simply to the technique of "attaching" regularly occurring functors and inflectional morphemes to contentives, e.g., (the + N), (is + V + ing). Patients who are capable of "chunking" this information will not overstress their syntactic processor after a period of practice with frequently used and predictable phrases. With regard to preposition usage, I have found that some patients find it easier to "tag" prepositions to the verb, e.g., (look + at), (go + to), than to the noun phrase, e.g., ([look] at + NP), ([go] to + NP). I respect such idiosyncratic "syntactic preferences" in my formulation of syntactic objectives.

In my experience, moderately severe Broca's aphasic patients have the most difficulty applying interphrasal syntactic rules. For this reason, I rarely attempt to teach complex syntactic forms, such as passive and conditional constructions, or embedding of relative clauses. Instead, I rely on concatenation, beginning with the conjunction "and" as in the constructions (N + V + O *and* N + V + O) or (NP + is + ADJ *and* NP + VP).

Finally, throughout the verbal expressive program, I stimulate writing skills, usually in the form of independent programs. Copying and spontaneous writing drills correspond directly to the syntactic forms being taught in the verbal program. In some patients, the recovery of writing surpasses the recovery of oral-verbal expression; in these cases, writing can be used to facilitate and reinforce oral-verbal syntactic remediation.

Visual-Spatial-Holistic Considerations

Prosodic contour.   The syllable is the minimal unit for prosodic reorganization. At this level, the cues are holistic motor patterns; treatment involves pairing action and vocalization. One strategy of this type is to pair facial expression with emotionally toned verbalizations to establish basic intonation patterns, e.g., surprise, negation, affirmation, interrogation. I also teach the patient to associate gross bodily movements with prosodic changes; movements of the arm in a vertical plane are associated with changes in stress, and movements in a horizontal plane are associated with changes in syllable duration and pause. Predictable movement patterns help to overcome initiation difficulty and help to re-establish control of prosody.

Phonologic form. At this level, the minimal unit is the word (or holophrase). Cues are holistic and static. I may teach the patient to use limb gestures to represent direction and locative relationships (e.g., here, there, up, down). I then introduce symbolic gestures. Initial signs are selected if they are concrete, meaningful, and easily executed. Signs are ideographic in the sense that they do not necessarily correspond to specific words or form classes, and many signs are pictographic as well. A second holistic-static reorganizing strategy involves the pairing of speech with printed words depicting highly imageable nouns, verbs, and adjectives. By manipulating rate of presentation, a "whole word" reading strategy can be encouraged. In the patient with severe dyslexia and/or limb apraxia, an alternative to gestures and whole word reading is the use of novel pictorial symbols. Novel symbols are not only holistic and static, but also nonphonetic and ideographic. Pairing of novel symbols with holophrastic utterances is designed to facilitate linguistic retrieval abilities.

Syntactic form. When words are combined into phrases and sentences, the specificity of language increases as does the complexity of syntactic rules. I begin training at this level by presenting frequently used phrases which may be rote memorized (e.g., let's go, time to go, wait for me, how are you?). The purpose of this transitional step is to establish phonologic-prosodic execution at the phrase level. This step is critical for stabilizing previously learned skills regarding stress, pause, duration, and tone.

Syntactic retraining *per se* begins with phrases and extends to kernel sentences and compound sentences. At this level of verbal reorganization, the cues are holistic, static, and sequential, while the response is phonologic, prosodic, sequential, and *rule-based*. Procedures at this stage are expansions of strategies established at earlier stages. This entails pairing speech with sequences of symbolic gestures, printed words (using whole word reading), and other ideograms (e.g., novel pictorial symbols). The repertoire of visual-holistic stimuli increases systematically with expansions in the rule-based syntactic forms selected for treatment.

Finally, to reorganize syntactic form, I use visual enhancement techniques. These include: (1) dictionary pronunciation symbols to represent phonetic distinctions and stress features, (2) punctuation marks to indicate interphrasal boundaries and intonational changes, and (3) phrase structure diagrams (tree diagrams) to enhance the patient's awareness of word order, form class distinctions, and the syntactic constraints within and across form classes.

CONCLUSIONS

The treatment described has been used eclectically with Broca's aphasic patients representing a wide variety of ages and etiologies. The treatment is ideally designed for aphasia of moderate or marked severity. I do not make this decision about "clinical severity" until (1) spontaneous recovery has been realized, and (2) the patient has been given the opportunity for treatment. The patient who acutely presents a profound oral-verbal deficit (e.g., undifferentiated nonfluent jargon or oral-verbal apraxia) may initially appear unsuited for an oral-verbal expressive program; periodic follow-up is recommended for such patients.

The early appearance of relatively preserved visual processing abilities is critical to long-term facilitation-reorganization potential. Visual-processing abilities of interest are: visual attention, visual scanning, visual comprehension of extralinguistic situational cues, visual comprehension of gestures and printed words, copying, writing, and gesturing ability. The patient's ability to *learn to use* spared functional systems in new and unprecedented ways can usually be determined after a relatively short period of therapy, i.e., one month of daily treatment, or the equivalent. I am always encouraged by "stimulability" within sessions, but I rely on measures of stability, retention, and generalization to help me make decisions about treatment efficacy and treatment (dis)continuation.

The success of treatment is highly individualized and depends both on the neuropsychological limitations of the patient and on the ability of the clinician to set realistic goals. The minimum goal for all patients is to provide a communication system that is effective, informative, and pragmatically flexible. In the Broca's aphasic patient of moderate severity, I strive to facilitate and reorganize phonologic-syntactic systems toward this end.

SELECTED REFERENCES

Caramazza, A., and Berndt, R. Semantic and syntactic processes in aphasia: A review of the literature. *Psychological Bulletin,* 1978, *85*:898–918.

Goodglass, H. Studies on the grammar of aphasics. In S. Rosenberg and J. Koplin (Eds.), *Developments in Applied Psycholinguistic Research.* New York: Macmillan, 1968.

Kean, M. The linguistic interpretation of aphasic syndromes: Agrammatism in Broca's aphasia, an example. *Cognition,* 1977, *5:*9–46.

Rosenbek, J. Treating apraxia of speech. In D. Johns (Ed.), *Clinical Management of Neurogenic Communicative Disorders.* Boston: Little, Brown, 1978 (pp. 191–242).

Rothi, L. and Horner, J. Theories of cortical function recovery with application to clinical neuropsychology. Journal of Clinical Neuropsychology, 1983. In press.

Acknowledgment: This chapter was funded in part by the Axe-Houghton Foundation, New York, New York.

CHAPTER TWO

TREATMENT OF WERNICKE'S APHASIA

Method of Judith L. Kennedy

"In Paris they simply stared when I spoke to them in French; I never did succeed in making those idiots understand their own language."

—*Mark Twain*

Because Mark Twain's condemnation did not extend to include the way they spoke their own language, we may assume that, indeed, his linguistic competence was greater than his performance. This axiom applies to all of us, including the majority of individuals with aphasic disorders. The only exception to the rule is the patient with Wernicke's aphasia. Employing a narrow definition of linguistic competence (comprehension) and performance (production), the Wernicke's aphasic is often equally impaired in both processes. This poses a dilemma to the clinician who has been taught to make use of intact, residual language competencies to facilitate change in both comprehension and production. And, as if this did not constitute enough of a challenge, the clinical picture of Wernicke's aphasia is often complicated by the presence of nonlanguage disorders in attention, awareness, and affect.

Specific techniques that have proved successful in treatment of all patients with Wernicke's aphasia and, thus, constitute a treatment approach have not been documented. My clinical experience together with the shared expertise of other clinicians has helped to formulate my belief that treatment of Wernicke's aphasia requires a flexible, eclectic, often experimental approach. The dictum, "If you think it will work, use it, and if it works, keep on using it," seems to be the clinical consensus.

A number of writers have expressed the belief that patients with Wernicke's aphasia are not candidates for treatment programs. I am not in agreement. All patients with communicative disorders are candidates for treatment, if we are able to alter and enlarge both our conception of treatment rationale and our repertoire of treatment techniques.

In this chapter, I will describe my approach to treating patients with Wernicke's aphasia. This approach is primarily directed toward those patients who have more severe language and behavioral disturbances. It reflects my clinical experience in an acute hospital setting.

ASSESSMENT FOR TREATMENT

A word or two about assessment. Assessment is implicit in any treatment design if one is to formulate methods and goals and to evaluate the effects of intervention. In a patient with aphasia, during the acute stages the clinical picture may often change rapidly and dramatically because of the disappearance of the widespread effect of a focal lesion (i.e., diaschisis). Ongoing assessment to document these changes in language function may sometimes be the major focus of "treatment" during this period.

My experience with assessment of Wernicke's aphasia in the early stages of hospitalization has taught me that I can spend my time more productively by making informal "clinical" assessments and counseling families and staff than by administering formal aphasia test batteries. Wernicke's aphasics with severe, and even moderate, language impairment may give minimal or no responses on formal testing. The clinician who is intent on obtaining PICA scores or Z scores on the BDAE may unintentionally aggravate behavioral symptomatology (paranoia and hostility) in the patient and cause confusion and consternation in staff and family members. Formal testing should be postponed until the patient has recovered to the extent that he is able to understand the purpose of the testing.

I look at three symptom areas in the Wernicke's aphasic to formulate clinical judgments about the nature and range of impairment. This allows me to make decisions about treatment intervention and provides a framework within which I can explain the patient's difficulties to the family and staff. Brief descriptions of symptom range and variability will be given.

Attention and Awareness

Many patients with Wernicke's aphasia have impaired ability to attend to and apprehend the rules of communication exchange. They exclusively assume the role of speaker and do not attend to cues generated by the receiver. Often these patients will continue speaking in response to minimal stimulation. In the most severely impaired, they may "converse" with tape recorders or the PA system (personal experience). In less severely impaired patients, this manifestation of inattention is still easily recognized by their "press of speech."

Most severely impaired Wernicke's aphasics are unable to recognize their own errors of speech. However, the preservation of self-monitoring behavior has been described in patients with severe comprehension problems (Lecours et al., 1981), suggesting that comprehension and awareness deficits do not always coexist in Wernicke's aphasia. Mildly impaired and recovering Wernicke's aphasics are often aware of their disordered speech and indicate this by their attitude and speech content.

Comprehension

The comprehension deficit of Wernicke's aphasia may be so severe that the patient is totally unable to comprehend spoken speech. More often, even patients with severe auditory processing deficits may be able to make use of paralinguistic cues in the environment to make appropriate responses to questions and commands, although inconsistently. Preservation of ability to follow whole body commands has also been documented in severely impaired patients. Patients with milder comprehension problems are able to follow simple commands and comprehend a great deal of conversational speech.

The variability of impairments is evident in the dissociation between oral langage and written language that is sometimes seen in patients. There is a subset of Wernicke's patients whose ability to use and comprehend written language is superior to their ability to use and comprehend oral language. Hier and Mohr (1977) describe a patient who was able to perform in writing the same naming tasks that he was unable to perform orally. The writing ability of some patients may therefore provide a better estimate of linguistic competence than their speaking performance. One of my patients who exhibited *no* ability to understand speech was able to understand written questions and follow some written directions. Comprehension should always be tested in both auditory and visual modalities.

Language Production

The language production disorder of Wernicke's aphasia is characterized by fluent paraphasic output. Verbal paraphasias are most frequent, although combinations of verbal and literal paraphasias are common. In its severest form, a mixture of both verbal and literal paraphasias results in an incomprehensible neologistic output. Because the paraphasic errors most often replace nouns, the resulting output may be incomprehensible to the listener. Predilection words (recurrent words) are not uncommon.

TREATMENT INTERVENTION FOR THE SEVERELY IMPAIRED PATIENT

Treatment of Wernicke's aphasics is dependent on the severity and range of these impairments. Patients who have little or no ability to recognize and comprehend auditory stimuli and who are not aware of their speech difficulties are not candidates for intensive and direct language treatment intervention. Intervention with these patients, instead, must emphasize improvement of communication. Since any communication exchange necessitates both a sender and a receiver of information, we need to improve our ability to both send and receive information from the aphasic patient. Lecours et al. (1981) state that Wernicke's aphasia is a "severe primary encoding difficulty in a speaker with a brain lesion and a secondary decoding difficulty in anyone listening." Because of the severity of the patient's deficits, the emphasis of treatment must be on the listener.

Focusing on the Clinician/Family as Senders of Information

The focus of this approach is to maximize the patient's ability to receive information by manipulating and altering the environment. These techniques are directed toward improving the patient's ability to attend to and comprehend information. They have not proved successful with all patients, nor have they all worked with any one patient. I have, however, found these techniques to be successful in changing behaviors in a large population of Wernicke's aphasics.

Techniques

Nonverbal "alerting" signals can be used by the clinician or family member to facilitate attentional set. Hand signals, e.g., a hand held in front of the patient to signify "stop and listen," or a finger held in front of the mouth to signify "quiet," are often effective in helping the patient to monitor and reduce his flow of speech. A slight turning away of the head may also be effective in signaling to the patient that his turn at speaking is over.

Gestures and demonstration coincident with verbal information should always be used. Some of the most severely auditorily impaired patients are able to make use of visual information. Positioning of the sender and recipient in a communication interaction is important. The patient as the receiver must be in a position to make full use of nonverbal information. The clinician/family can increase the likelihood of a patient's comprehending the intent, if not the full meaning, of communication by stressing extralinguistic cues, e.g., body posture, voice intonation, facial expressions. Attempting to "get information into the brain" means using whatever seems to work. The spouse of one of my patients, when all else failed, resorted to making simple sketches of objects and actions to convey information. I have since used this technique with other patients and have encouraged other family members, who have used it with success.

Another method, alluded to earlier, is the use of written information. This technique, when successful, may have impact on all three symptom areas: attention, comprehension, and output. The patient is alerted to the sender's intention to communicate. The written information may activate residual visually based language competence. It may also serve to elicit more correct and appropriate output.

One of my patients with severe Wernicke's aphasia was able to understand enough written information to respond to questions such as "How are you? What is your name? Do you have children?" and to appreciate the meaning of "Time to eat. Time for bed." She was unable to comprehend the same information when it was spoken to her.

Other techniques focus on maximizing input through the auditory channel. They are useful for all patients who have auditory processing difficulties. Extraneous background noise should be eliminated with Wernicke's patients. They often have difficulty focusing on meaningful auditory stimuli when the PA system, physicians' rounds at the next bedside, T.V., and radio are competing for attention. Multiple, simultaneous conversations are also difficult for these patients. Even those with mild, residual difficulty in auditory processing continue to favor one-on-one or small group interactions.

The use of verbal alerters, e.g., the patient's name, may help to orient his attention to the fact that communication will follow. The rate at which this information is given (rate of speech and the use of intraphrase pauses) does influence comprehension. Patients with auditory deficits require significantly longer periods of time to process auditory information. Although this fact is self-evident to most clinicians, families and staff are often unaware of the impact. I have found it necessary not only to restate this precept over and over again to families and staff, but to model it as well.

Judicious use of repetition improves comprehension in Wernicke's aphasics who have residual auditory comprehension. I use repetition sparingly with the more severely impaired. With these patients, it seems to have little effect and may easily "overload" the auditory system. When I do use repetition as a facilitator, I have also found it helpful to use alerters such as "Let me say it again," or, "Listen."

Other variables which can be manipulated by the speaker and which affect the patient's comprehension are (1) increasing the redundancy of the message, e.g., "Show me the fork [the one that you eat with]," (2) decreasing syntactic complexity (i.e., using simple declarative sentences), (3) selection of vocabulary (i.e., using high-frequency, short, meaningful words), and (4) decreasing length of utterance. These should all be considered with the Wernicke's aphasic.

Focusing on the Clinician/Family as Receivers of Information

In addition to becoming more aware of how they give information to the patient, the clinician and family need to become more receptive to the patient's communication. Family members are usually more adept at doing this than are other individuals involved with the patient (including the clinician). By virtue of their long, close association, they have learned to recognize and interpret the patient's nonverbal behaviors, i.e., facial expression, vocal parameters, eye contact, body posture. Other family members and caregivers need to be reminded that the patient's nonverbal communication is capable of conveying considerable information.

Since "yes/no" responses may be particularly difficult for these patients, other indicators of response should be looked for. One patient consistently answered "yes" to every question that was asked. To questions that required a "no" response, he would characteristically repeat a word or part of the question in a quite incredulous tone of voice. By distinguishing this pattern of response, we were better able to ascertain what the patient understood as well as interpret the patient's communication.

Coincident with working on interpretation of the patient's nonverbal communication with the family, we also need to encourage patients to use nonverbal forms of communication and the family to accept them. I have not succeeded in teaching Wernicke's patients to use manual signals and gestures systematically, although some clinicians have reported success. I have, however, with some success, encouraged patients' attempts at writing and even drawing. Although these tasks are often difficult for the Wernicke's patient, they may provide enough additional information to facilitate the intention of communication. A statement and request—"I'm not sure what you are saying. Can you show me what you mean?''—may prompt the patient to search through his own repertoire of communication strategies, and may result in a gesture or action that succeeds in augmenting communication (e.g., reaching into his pocket for a wallet, or going to find a nurse or doctor).

I have also spent time with families in helping them to understand and interpret the disordered output of the patient. Predilection words and utterances can be very confusing to families and caregivers. Some examples will illustrate. One patient in the early stages of his recovery constantly interjected "Why?" into his conversation. This would frequently result in lengthy explanations from family and caregiver alike, which the patient neither wanted nor understood, and which contributed to a true conversational cacophony. Both family and caregivers needed to be informed that the patient was not requesting information. Another patient, an attorney, frequently peppered his conversation with legal terms. The family, initially assuming that he was conversing about his law practice, wanted to bring in information about pending legal cases. The family needed to understand that the patient's choice of words (predilection words) did not carry one-to-one correspondence.

I have also counseled families of some Wernicke's patients to pay more attention to the parts of speech that typically carry less information than other parts, and to try to decipher meaning from the whole of the utterance. Because neologisms and paraphasias typically replace nouns, other parts of speech—i.e., adjectives, adverbs, and verbs—may be retrieved and used appropriately. One patient was able to convey that he wanted "a cup of coffee and hold the cream and sugar" with the following utterances: "I want a black coker, with a pure . . . and don't put any burnee on it." By ignoring the paraphasic errors and paying attention to the "gestalt" of the utterances, it was not difficult to understand what the patient was communicating.

TREATMENT INTERVENTION FOR THE LESS SEVERELY IMPAIRED PATIENT

As patients improve, they become candidates for traditional treatment programs that focus on improving auditory comprehension and verbal expression. It is at this point that both standardized tests and intensive, repetitive, and controlled auditory stimulation can be used with favorable results.

Most Wernicke's patients will benefit from a well-designed program to treat auditory comprehension. Implementation of an auditory comprehension program presupposes careful and thorough assessment of the patient's auditory capabilities and disabilities. Assessment for treatment will take into account (1) the type and severity of the comprehension deficit, (2) the variables (linguistic, timing, contextual) that can be manipulated to effect changes in comprehension, and (3) the communicative conditions under which comprehension is either enhanced or diminished.

Standardized measurements will provide data on the type and severity of the comprehension deficit, but will be of little use in providing information about the variables and conditions that may alter patients' comprehension. It is up to the clinician to collect this information in a systematic way, to incorporate it into the treatment design, and to share it with the patient and family.

Apart from the work on auditory comprehension that patients and clinicians do together in therapy, there is work to be done outside of therapy. The patient and family, together with the clinician, can identify communicative situations that are difficult, explore the possible causes, and begin to make modifications that allow the patient to function best with his auditory capabilities. I have found this exploration to be beneficial to patients and families. One of our mildly impaired patients was disturbed by his inability to follow the television news programs. With further discussion, it became clear that the news program format (multiple news stories and rapid change of topics) coupled with the fast speaking rate of the newscasters did not allow him sufficient time to process the information. He devised the strategies of watching both the early and late evening news broadcasts, having his wife read the newspaper to him, and daily discussing news events with his family and friends. Another patient had always socialized with his large group of friends in front of the television. After his stroke, he found these occasions to be more frustrating than fun, and complained that the conversation "moved too fast" and "was tiring." It was suggested to the patient that he rotate his friends to limit the size of the group and turn off the T.V. By eliminating excessive competing and background auditory stimuli, he found that he again enjoyed the visits.

Several of the language behaviors that characterize Wernicke's aphasia can be capitalized on by incorporating them into the treatment program. Identifying the patient's repertoire of predilection words and recurrent words will often provide a core of language material for repetition, identification, oral reading, and reading recognition tasks. This often provides a starting point in therapy for working on verbal expression. We began work on repetition and oral reading with the attorney by using, almost exclusively, his litany of legal terms. These were the words and expressions he used frequently in conversation, and they proved to be the easiest for him to produce volitionally (either by repetition or oral reading). Once this task was learned and performed adequately, we were able to introduce more appropriate and desirable lexical material.

The tendency for patients with Wernicke's aphasia to produce copious, often circumlocutionary speech can also be used to advantage in therapy. Since the act of naming in itself frequently produces a more disordered output, I rarely work on direct naming tasks. Instead, I work on the "act of description" with patients. I ask them to describe a lexical item by discussing parameters such as function, size, and color. The act of description often elicits more meaningful speech from the patient and, consequently, more information for the listener. This activity can be modeled for the patient by both the clinician and the family. When used judiciously so as not to encourage excessive speech, this technique can be helpful in directing access to lexical forms which may be relatively intact (e.g., verbs, adjectives). This technique is widely used with the anomic patient to teach him to circumvent his naming difficulties by using description and explanation, and may be just as successful with Wernicke's aphasics who have underlying anomic deficits.

SUMMARY

Treating the impaired communication of Wernicke's aphasia broadly challenges the therapeutic armamentarium of the aphasia clinician. The multiplicity and variability of symptoms do not easily lend themselves to the use of a "cookbook" approach to treatment. Instead, the clinician must assume the role of the "creative chef" who by virtue of training and experience is able to concoct, simmer, and taste (i.e., formulate, carry through, and evaluate) many variations on the recipe for treatment. When we are able to do this and effect desired changes in patient and family behavior as a result of our intervention, we can truly savor the sweet taste of success.

SELECTED REFERENCES

Hecaen, H., and Albert, M. *Human Neuropsychology*. New York: John Wiley and Sons, 1978.

Hier, D., and Mohr, J.P., Incongruous oral and written naming. *Brain and Language*, 1977, *4*, 115–126.

Lecours, A.R., Osborn, E., Travis, L., Rouillon, F., and Lavallee-Huyhn, G. Jargons. In J. W. Brown (Ed.), *Jargonaphasia*. New York: Academic Press, 1981.

Marshall, R. Heightening auditory comprehension for aphasic patients. In R. Chapey (Ed.), *Language Intervention Strategies in Adult Aphasia*. Baltimore: Williams and Wilkins, 1981.

Martin, A.D. Therapy with the jargonaphasic. In J. W. Brown (Ed.) *Jargonaphasia*. New York: Academic Press, 1981.

Schuell, H., Jenkins, J. J., and Jimenez-Pabon, E. *Aphasia in Adults: Diagnosis, Prognosis and Treatment*. New York: Harper and Row, 1964.

CHAPTER THREE

TREATMENT OF GLOBAL APHASIA

Method of Michael Collins

Among the aphasias, none has so shattering an impact on life as global aphasia. The term, and its historical predecessors, "irreversible aphasic syndrome," and "total aphasia," suggests a disorder so pervasive that the ability to receive and transmit messages is hopelessly, irretrievably lost. Implicit in that statement is the suggestion that treatment will have little impact on recovery. Although that bleak prospect may be true in some cases, it is also true that many of these patients recover considerable communicative ability.

There is probably at least a triad of global aphasias: acute, chronic, and evolutional. Acute global aphasia is often seen in the very early stages of recovery, but may be transient. In evolutional global aphasia, a distinct subtype (often Broca's aphasia) will emerge, not uncommonly after months or even years. In chronic global aphasia, profound deficits persist in all communicative modalities despite the healing effect of time. Early identification of these subgroups may be possible only in retrospect, or only after a period of unavailing treatment, but several characteristics seem to differentiate those destined to become chronic global aphasic patients from other members of the triad:

1. There is severe depression of communicative ability across all modalities, and no single communicative modality is strikingly better than another.

2. Visual, nonverbal problem-solving abilities are often severely depressed, and are usually compatible with language performance.

3. Recovery will be agonizingly slow; most traditional stimulation procedures will be inappropriate and their effects often negligible; learning curves on even the simplest tasks will be ephemeral.

Despite rigorous examination of formal and informal test results, I, and other clinicians, am handicapped by uncertain prognosis, and my treatment in the early stages of recovery reflects this uncertainty. Thus, my goals for all patients in the first few crucial weeks of treatment are similar: (1) modify the equivocal response, (2) institute a diagnostic treatment program to reduce the uncertainty of prognosis, (3) identify appropriate treatment candidates, (4) justify my treatment decisions, and (5) establish a treatment program in which the patient's, the family's, and my goals coincide.

This chapter is devoted to the treatment of the chronic, globally aphasic patient who remains speechless. The experienced clinician will recognize the signs of emergence from that condition, and modify treatment accordingly. The focus of my treatment is on total communication, but I have not found direct speech drill to be efficacious, and it is not discussed in this chapter. If useful speech emerges at any point, it is accepted enthusiastically and incorporated into this program.

THE EQUIVOCAL RESPONSE

Globally aphasic patients understand more than they can express. While some of their messages may not be confusing, their "yes" and "no" responses are often equivocal and present a more significant barrier to communication than impaired comprehension. My immediate objective is to establish unequivocal yes and no responses in verbal or nonverbal form. I follow the procedure framed in Table 1 for shaping and stabilizing the response, and focus on getting clear signals in and clear signals out. Stabilization of "yes" and "no" is enhanced by playing the card game "21." Patients enjoy playing the game, and, of equal importance, a clear, unequivocal response is required to "Do you want another card?" Additional benefits are the social interaction and the stimulation provided by the calculations.

When the response is stable, I baseline responses to a series of

TABLE 1 Shaping and Stabilizing Response

Shaping the Yes and No Resonse
  1. Physically assist the patient with 5 repetitions of yes (head nod), then no (side to side head movements) while clinician says the word.
  2. Alternate gestured yes, then no, with physical assistance while clinician says the word. Pause approximately 5 seconds between responses.
  3. Request gestured responses to simple unambiguous questions while clinician assists with gestures and says the word.

Stabilizing the Response
  1. Request 5 repetitions of gestured yes, then no. Facilitate with physical or verbal cues if required.
  2. Request alternating yes, then no, at approximately 5 second intervals, facilitating if required.
  3. Request gestured responses to simple questions, facilitating if required.

20 simple, usually biographical, questions and select ten of these for treatment. The other ten questions are not treated, but are used to measure the effects of generalization. I measure both stimulus sets at regular intervals. When performance on the treated set reaches 80 to 90 percent correct, and that level is sustained for several sessions, I baseline, then treat the second set of ten questions, and continue to baseline both sets. This is essentially a modified withdrawal design, but there are numerous single-case designs for measuring the effects of treatment. These designs are powerful because they insist on controlled-stimulus conditions, force one to specify treatment goals, insist on careful observation and recording of behaviors, allow both clinician and patient to observe meaningful changes in communicative behaviors, enable clinicians to determine adequacy or inadequacy of specific treatments, and document the effects of treatment.

TREATMENT FORMAT

Most of my treatment sessions follow a similar format: An introduction, in which we discuss time, place, weather, and similar topics in which I assume most of the communicative burden; review and measure easier, previously treated tasks; introduce new stimuli or tasks; and a decompression period, emphasizing the patient's most successful tasks, conversation, or card playing.

In these early stages of recovery, length of treatment sessions will be determined by the patient's endurance, but are generally no more than one-half hour twice daily. I expand treatment time as the patient's endurance improves.

This format, or a similar one in which patients experience early success, moves gradually toward tasks that tax abilities and provide for a successful denouement. How one provides detail for this framework will depend upon the patient's severity, interests, progress, and the hierarchy of task difficulty developed from formal and informal test results.

My primary objective is to help the patient reach a level of independent communication. Thus, my treatment sessions are not always rigidly structured, but, like the Sears Tower or the design for a Navajo rug, bend when it is appropriate. Nevertheless, I devote a portion of each session to a hierarchy of tasks that fall under the rubric "stimulation," such as those provided by Duffy (1981). Hierarchies such as these provide a foundation for communication, much as the binnacle does for the compass, but they are hollow until the clinician fills them with adequate stimuli. To ensure that the stimuli are adequate, the clinician must be thoroughly familiar with the general principles underlying stimulus presentation. Excellent summaries of these principles can be found in Duffy (1981). Salience of stimuli may be the most important of these.

Salience of Stimuli

Salient stimuli are those that are striking or conspicuous, but salience varies among individuals. A Brahms sonata may not be salient to a Willie Nelson fan, nor a sandhi to an electrician. Several classes of stimuli appear to be more salient than others to globally aphasic patients. Brand names, for example, can be strikingly effective. They may, in fact, be used as preliminary stimuli in an auditory program, as warm-ups, or as adjuncts. Familiar topics, for example, words and activities related to hobbies and occupations, family names, and geographic place names are often salient stimuli for globally aphasic patients. Whenever possible, I use stimuli that are maximally salient.

Total Communication

Total communication for the globally aphasic patient might be viewed as an extension of what normal communicators utilize when available vocabulary fails to convey their ideas adequately. Drawing, gesturing, and writing are often used as adjuncts to spoken communication, and may at times be more powerful. Total communication emphasizes the use—sometimes simultaneously, sometimes concurrently, and sometimes consecutively—of every available, or potentially available, means of communication, including communication boards.

In the early stages of treatment, total communication requires arduous, didactic instruction in the use of one or more of the modes I have outlined for the yes/no response, and a significant portion of each treatment session is devoted to gestural communication as a prelude to total communication.

Gestural Communication

In early sessions, I assess spontaneous gestural ability informally in conversation; formally, in response to pictured or auditory stimuli;

and imitatively. If any gestures are intact, even if they are idiosyncratic, they are retained as part of the core. I select approximately ten gesturable actions, for example, eat, drink, smoke, listen. I use real objects when pantomime does not elicit the response. I expand the core when all ten gestures have been acquired, and maintain them by periodic assessment and retraining for the recidivists.

A general outline for this gestural program is shown in Table 2. I begin with one gesture, presenting both spoken and gestured stimuli, until that gesture is intact, then expand to two gestures, alternating between the two with fewer repetitions of each until the patient can alternate gestures successively through the final step. I add a third gesture and repeat the process until all three gestures are firmly established. I add gestures in this way as competence is demonstrated.

Once the patient has learned several gestures, uses them in response to questions, and recognizes the need for them, they are incorporated into a program of total communication.

Gestures are not limited to their use as emblems. Pointing, for example, is probably best described as an illustrator which, when used alone, conveys a message succinctly. When accompanied by verbal or nonverbal facilitators, such as facial expression, speech, or writing, it illuminates the message.

POINTING

Pointing is an integral part of total communication and can be used to convey a primary message and to impart attributes of an object or concept. The first step in incorporating contextual pointing in a program of total communication is to establish a clear, unequivocal gesture. Initially, accuracy of response is not nearly as important

TABLE 2 Strengthening the Gestural Response

1. *Clinician* gestures and says word simultaneously.
2. *Clinician* says word, clinician and patient gesture simultaneously (clinician assistance with gesture may be required).
3. *Patient* imitates gesture.
4. *Patient* imitates gesture after enforced delay.
5. *Patient* gestures in response to auditory stimulus.
6. *Patient* gestures in response to auditory stimulus after enforced delay.
7. *Patient* gestures in response to written stimulus.
8. *Patient* gestures in response to written stimulus after enforced delay.
9. *Patient* writes word in response to gestural and auditory stimulus.
10. *Patient* gestures in response to appropriate question.

as establishing a clear response. At this stage, I may ask the patient to point to one object, or pictured object, with no foil. If the response is inadequate, I have the patient imitate my gesture until it is intact. As response adequacy increases, I add one foil, and drill each step until adequacy is achieved. Next, the stimulus field is expanded by asking the patient to point to objects in the room, imitating my gesture when necessary. Finally, I ask the patient to look at a series of realistic, colored pictures, first pointing to objects in the picture I've identified, then point to corresponding items in the room. I employ a similar procedure for conveying attributes such as color, by having the patient point to objects of the same color as the target.

For some patients, even the most severe, playing cards are the most salient of objects. I use card matching and identification tasks to stabilize the pointing response, and I often use this task as a warm-up exercise. Many patients tolerate four foils, but the cards should be maximally differentiated, for example, ace of spades, king of clubs, nine of diamonds, and seven of hearts. Pointing drill can also be expanded to include drill with a communication board.

COMMUNICATION BOARDS

A simple communication board containing pictured objects and actions of daily living can be an effective method of communicating for some patients. I supplement these pictures with large print words when necessary and where appropriate; I haven't found "alphabet" boards, nor boards that contain only the printed word, to be effective. Some patients, however, benefit from the combination of word and picture.

When I train patients in the use of such boards, I begin by limiting the field to no more than one foil, and expand the foils to include the whole board when the patient can manage it. Initially, I use contextually redundant stimuli, e.g., "Show me the bed—the one you sleep in," move to less redundant stimuli, "Show me the one you sleep in," and then "Show me the bed," imposing approximately five-second delays at each step. Still limiting the array to items we've worked on in this way, I ask the patient to use the board for expression, e.g., "Which one would you point to if you were tired?" and expand this core as the patient improves. Many patients will never use a board functionally, but many can use it to supplement other communicative modalities.

WRITING

Writing will never be a functional, independent modality, but an approximation of a verb or noun can be persuasive. Part of each treatment session, or at least part of one of the two daily sessions, is devoted to writing. Initially, I confine drill to copying, with assistance if necessary. All stimuli are simple, meaningful, salient, and maximally differentiated. The sequence I follow is listed in Table 3.

DRAWING

When words or gestures fail, many of us rely on simple illustrations. Pictures probably aren't worth a thousand words, but may be worth a precious few. Many globally aphasic patients, despite severe visual deficits, retain some artistic ability, albeit often crude. I don't teach drawing in any structured sense, but I encourage it in the sending of messages, and often shape the patient's drawing or have him copy mine.

COMBINING MODALITIES FOR TOTAL COMMUNICATION

Like the man who, when asked if he could read the sign right over there, said "I can't read and write at the same time," most of us can be stressed by simultaneous stimuli. The globally aphasic patient is uniquely susceptible to the confusion caused by too much stimulation. Some combinations, however, appear to be better than others. The combination of lexical, gestural, and auditory stimuli is a particularly powerful input, and gesture, including pointing and writing, are particularly effective outputs for the globally aphasic patient.

Once I have demonstrated that each of the components can be

TABLE 3 Writing Drill Sequence

1. Tracing of single words (assist if necessary)
2. Copying of single words
3. Brief presentation of auditory and lexical stimulus, written response
4. Brief presentation of auditory and lexical stimulus, imposed delay (5-15 seconds), written response
5. Writing to dictation
6. Writing to pictured presentation
7. Writing in response to question, e.g. "What would you say if you were thirsty?"

used in relative independence, I try to weave a communicative fabric using two or more of these components. The key to that, I think, involves the training that has already occurred: establish the conditions for communication, provide a communicative umbrella that protects the patient from the effects of failure, and make treatment as meaningful and relevant to the patient's life as possible.

Step 1 in this program of total communication involves the teaching of independent skills and encouraging their use in natural communication.

Step 2 is the culmination of those efforts, in which the patient and clinician utilize these skills to communicate. In this step, the patient is provided with pencil, paper, and communication board. These are treated as natural extensions of the communicative process, and placed for easy access. Using realistic, colored cards that depict only one clear action, I ask the patient to describe the action in any or all of the modalities open to him. Responses that communicate the action are accepted. I don't require "accurate" responses, but responses that communicate. When the response communicates, my response is a modeling of the patient's response. When the patient fails to communicate, I present a communicative response in each modality open to me, pause, and ask the patient again to communicate that action. As competence improves, the vocabulary core is expanded. When he can communicate approximately ten of these actions, I engage the patient in a more natural communicative exchange. The ten cards are randomized and divided between the patient and myself. In turn, each of us turns a card over, and attempts to communicate the action portrayed on the card. The patient is required to signal his understanding of the message either by replicating my message or affirming that message in another modality.

In Step 3, the patient's spouse, near friend, or relative is actively involved in treatment, and trained in that patient's total communication skills if possible. My role then becomes one of facilitator.

Step 4, which is often the final step in this program, revolves around themes that incorporate the patient's family, holidays, vacation, travel, avocations, and current events. In these sessions, I ask the patient to identify one or two themes for discussion, or I select a theme. As the theme is developed, central and related descriptors are incorporated in as natural a manner as possible. If the topic is fishing, for example, I might begin by presenting the major topic, and follow by asking the patient to tell me the largest fish he's caught, what kind, where, and similar information.

Again, no response is "inaccurate," but some replies are more communicative than others. All are reinforced or modeled, and extensions of the theme follow. The burden of communication is on the clinician, but in subsequent sessions I try to transfer as much of that burden to the patient as he will accept. Most patients accept the challenge, and respond to the level of their communicative abilities.

HOMEWORK

Homework for the globally aphasic patient need not, and should not, be busy work. I use homework as an extension of my treatment for total communication. If there is a willing partner at home, and the procedure does not disrupt relationships, I train the partner in these techniques, and ask him/her to provide at least daily treatment sessions. If the partner is reluctant, or the atmosphere not conducive to this approach, all patients are assigned single words, usually nouns, family names, biographical place names, and verbs relevant to daily living and current themes; they are asked to copy them several times a day. This written work is reviewed, shaped, and incorporated into the next session.

CONCLUSION

Treatment for the globally aphasic patient will be protracted, and will require enduring patience, understanding, and cooperation from patient, family, and clinician. In part because we provide these supports, patients will express their dignity and their concerns despite ravaged communicative skills, loss of their accustomed control of their environment, and the daily indignities suffered in a verbal world. By caring and communicating, we can extend the patient's communicative lifeline.

SELECTED REFERENCES

Chester, S. and Egolf, D. Nonverbal communication and aphasia therapy. *Rehabilitation Literature,* 1974, *35*:231–233.

Davis, G. and Wilcox, M. Incorporating parameters of natural conversation in aphasia treatment. In R. Chapey (Ed.), *Language Intervention Strategies in Adult Aphasia.* Baltimore: Williams and Wilkins, 1981.

Duffy, J. Schuell's stimulation approach to rehabilitation. In R. Chapey (Ed.), *Language Intervention Strategies in Adult Aphasia.* Baltimore: Williams and Wilkins, 1981.

Sarno, M. and Levita, E. Some observations on the nature of recovery in global aphasia after stroke. *Brain and Language,* 1981, *13*:1-12.

Towey, M. and Pettit, J. Improving communication competence in global aphasia. in R. Brookshire (Ed.), *Clinical Aphasiology: Conference Proceedings, 1980.* Minneapolis, MN: BRK Publishers, 1980.

CHAPTER FOUR

TREATMENT OF ANOMIC APHASIA

Method of Craig W. Linebaugh

Anomic aphasia is a specific aphasic syndrome marked by a pattern of language behaviors for which the treatment approaches to be described in this chapter are intended. The primary deficit in anomic aphasia is disruption of the process of word retrieval. The severity of this deficit may range from extreme difficulty in retrieving lexical items on all tasks to relatively mild deficits manifest only in conversational speech.

The verbal output of anomic aphasic patients is essentially fluent and frequently includes verbal paraphasias and circumlocutions. Repetition is good, and auditory comprehension is generally only mildly impaired. Impairments of reading and writing range considerably in severity. In this chapter, only approaches to the treatment of the word retrieval deficit will be discussed. Therapy for impairments of other language abilities are described elsewhere.

Because of the range of severity of the word-retrieval deficits encountered in anomic aphasia, two different treatment approaches will be described. The first involves cueing hierarchies; I employ it with patients with moderate to severe word-retrieval deficits. The second, referred to as Lexical Focus, I use for mild disturbances.

MODERATE-SEVERE ANOMIC APHASIA: CUEING HIERARCHIES

Rationale

Cueing is an effective and widely used technique in aphasia rehabilitation. It appears, however, that cues are often employed in what is essentially a random, trial-and-error fashion. The cueing hierarchy approach was designed to employ an individual patient's residual skills and responsiveness to specific types of cues in a more systematic manner. This approach is particularly suited to the anomic aphasic patient in that it seeks to make optimal use of his preserved repetition and auditory comprehension, and residual reading and writing abilities.

Three principles have guided the development of the cueing hierarchy approach. First, it is my belief that the patient's recovery is best served by eliciting the desired response with a minimum of external facilitation or cueing. That is, the stimulus should be no more powerful than necessary to elicit a given response. The second principle is a modification of the concept of stimulus fading. It advocates that the stimulus required to elicit a given response should be faded immediately upon elicitation of the response, rather than over time, in accordance with criteria based on a group of responses. In cueing hierarchies, this is achieved by eliciting the response with successively less powerful cues immediately following its accurate production. The third principle calls for the development and use of internal facilitators or self-generated cues by the patient.

Construction of Cueing Hierarchies

It is essential that one recognize that the relative stimulus power (that is, the probability that a given cue will elicit the desired response) of various types of cues varies among patients. Therefore, I develop the cueing hierarchy to be employed for each patient individually. Every hierarchy, however, contains certain types of cues.

The first, or least powerful, cue in any hierarchy is referred to as a "task orientation cue." In a naming task, for example, I may simply ask "What's this called?" The next one or two cues are designed to elicit self-generated cues on the part of the patient. The type of self-generated cue sought is dependent on the patient's residual skills and the relative effectiveness of such cues. Thus, I may ask one patient to "show me what you do with it," if gesture is an effective facilitator for him. Another patient, whose graphic skills are relatively intact, may be asked to write the word or its first letter.

The next group of cues are various external facilitators that have been found to be effective for the patient. Table 1 lists the types of cues that I have found to be effective with a number of patients. These cues are placed in the hierarchy in order of increasing stimulus power. I develop this sequence of cues by assessing their

TABLE 1   Types of Cues

Gesture
Association
Description
Function
Sentence completion
Phonemic
Graphic

TABLE 2   A Cueing Hierarchy

7. What's this called?
6. Can you tell me what you do with it?
5. Can you show me what you do with it
4. You write with it. It's a . . .
3. You write with a ballpoint____.
2. You write with a [p]____.
1. Say *pen*.

relative power for a given patient on a series of items over three therapy sessions.

The final cue in any hierarchy is one that will elicit the desired response with essentially 100 percent probability. For the anomic aphasic patient with preserved repetition, this is a cue to imitation. Table 2 illustrates a typical cueing hierarchy for word retrieval.

Stimulus Items

I select 20 stimulus items (e.g., objects, pictures) to which the patient will respond on the basis of functionality and their relevance to the patient's environment (both immediate and that of projected disposition) and interests. The stimuli may be designed to elicit whatever length of response (e.g., single word, phrase, sentence, descriptive narrative) is appropriate for the patient. Care must be taken to ensure that the stimuli are compatible with the cues being employed.

Therapy Procedure

The 20 stimulus items are divided into two sets of 10, which are used in alternate therapy sessions. Initially, I present each stimulus along with the task orientation cue. Successively more powerful cues are presented until the patient produces an acceptable response. When this occurs, I present the cues in order of decreasing stimulus power, ending with the task orientation cue. For those cues designed to elicit a self-generated cue, I require the patient to produce the self-generated cue (modeling it if necessary), as well as the response. If the patient fails to respond accurately to any of the successively less powerful cues, I reverse the order of presentation until he again produces an acceptable response. Once again, the order of presentation is reversed, leading to the initial cue. This order reversal is done only once per stimulus, even if the patient is unable to return to the initial cue.

Scoring

The order number of the cue at which the patient first produces an acceptable response is recorded and serves as his score for that item. The need for reversal of the order of presentation and the number of the cue at which an acceptable response is again produced is also noted. Valuable information may also be obtained by noting the patient's response to each cue, but this is rather cumbersome without resorting to use of a separate score sheet for each treatment session. The mean cueing level, that is, the mean number of the cues at which acceptable responses were elicited for a series of stimuli, may also be of importance in evaluating treatment efficacy.

Criteria

I employ three types of criteria for this procedure. The first, response criterion, specifies what is an acceptable response for a given stimulus. The second, task completion criterion, specifies an acceptable level of performance and serves as an indication of response stability. For the cueing hierarchy approach, I usually specify task completion criteria as an acceptable response (as defined in the response criterion) on 80 to 90 percent of the stimuli to either the task orientation cue or a cue designed to elicit a self-generated cue. These levels of stimulus power are considered acceptable in that they can be employed in functional communication. The use of a more powerful cue requires that the listener already know the intended response.

I refer to the third criterion as the task modification criterion. This is an indication of plateau in the patient's performance short of the task criterion. I express this criterion as an increment in the mean cueing level over a predetermined number of therapy sessions. Thus, if the patient does not show at least a one-point change in the mean cueing level over five sessions, his performance is re-evaluated, and the task modified as indicated. This may include replacing or eliminating ineffective cues or particularly difficult items. Also, if the patient consistently responds accurately to the task orientation cue on six of the 10 items in either of the sets, half of these items are replaced.

Generalization

In addition to the 20 stimulus items used in therapy, a third set of 10 stimuli are used to measure generalization. These stimuli are presented every fifth to tenth session, depending on how frequently the patient is seen. For this set, the cues are presented only in order of increasing stimulus power. I have found that gains in word retrieval attained by using cueing hierarchies have generalized well to untrained items.

MILD ANOMIC APHASIA: LEXICAL FOCUS

Rationale

The word-retrieval deficit of the mild anomic aphasic patient most often manifests itself in three ways. Two of these manifestations, inappropriate pauses and circumlocutions, represent potentially effective compensatory strategies. I frequently work with patients in order to make their use of these strategies as productive and efficient as possible. The third manifestation of a mild word-retrieval deficit is verbal paraphasia, and it is the nature of these "errors" of word retrieval that underlies the treatment approach I call "lexical focus."

Verbal paraphasias are the substitution of a related word for the intended word. Frequently, the word actually produced lies within the same superordinate category as does the intended word. For example, a patient may substitute *fork* for *spoon;* both words lie in the category of silverware. Psycholinguistic research has provided evidence that lexicon is organized along several dimensions. Among these appear to be superordinate categories based on semantic features. A verbal paraphasia then suggests that the patient has gained access to the appropriate superordinate category, but has selected the wrong lexical item from that category. The purpose of lexical focus therapy, therefore, is to increase the patient's lexical agility; that is, to enable him to more efficiently scan the lexical items in a given category and select the desired word.

Stimuli

The stimuli I use in lexical focus consist of superordinate categories of various widths. Category width refers to the number of lexical items contained in a given category. Currently, I employ categories of three widths. First-order categories are those of the greatest width, i.e., they contain the greatest number of lexical items. Second-order categories are those containing approximately one-half to two-thirds of the items within a given first-order category. Third-order categories, in turn, contain one-half to two-thirds of the items within a given second-order category. Table 3 lists several of the sets of categories I employ.

TABLE 3 Categories for Lexical Focus

First-order	Second-order	Third-order
Fruits & Vegetables	Fruits Vegetables	Citrus fruits Berries Green vegetables Yellow vegetables
Furniture	Living room furniture Bedroom furniture	Furniture you sit on

Clothing	Men's
	Women's
		Clothes you'd
		  pack for a trip
		  to Alaska in
		  winter

Sports	Played with a ball
	Not played with a
	  ball
		Played with a
		  racket
		Water sports

Therapy Procedure

In the lexical focus procedure, I instruct the patient to name as many items as he can in a given category. Four or five categories may be presented, either as a block or at various times during a therapy session. Lexical focus begins with first-order categories. Second- and third-order categories are presented on meeting predetermined criteria to be discussed.

Each set of categories moves at its own pace. Thus, in a given session, I may present two first-order categories, two second-order categories, and a third-order category. I avoid presenting a second- or third-order category immediately following its own superordinate category.

The patient is permitted to continue naming items in a given category until 20 seconds elapse with no accurate response. When this occurs, if the patient has not met criterion, a "search strategy" is provided. A search strategy is not a cue for a specific item in the category. Rather, it is a device to aid the patient in organizing his search for appropriate items. For example, for the category of furniture, the patient may be instructed to think about the furniture in his own home. For vegetables, he may be asked to imagine walking through the produce section of a supermarket. As therapy progresses, I frequently require the patient to develop his own search strategies. Indeed, many patients begin to do so on their own and employ them spontaneously.

Scoring

Scoring for lexical focus consists of counting the number of items produced in 15-second intervals. Note that the elapsed time between accurate responses must be monitored so that a search strategy can be provided following 20 unproductive seconds. The provision of a search strategy and the number of items produced afterward should also be recorded. I have found recording the patient's actual responses helpful in determining his spontaneous use of associations and search strategies.

Criteria

I employ the following critera for lexical focus: first-order categories: 10 items in 60 seconds; second-order categories: 7 items in

60 seconds; third-order categories: 4 items in 60 seconds. If a patient's performance plateaus at "criterion-2 items" for 3 sessions on a given first- or second-order category, the next narrower category may be presented. If performance plateaus at less than "criterion-2 items" for 3 sessions, I replace the category with a new first-order category.

Generalization

I assess generalization of gains on lexical focus in two ways. One is by periodic administration of the "animal-naming" subtest of the Boston Diagnostic Aphasia Examination. This, of course, precludes using animals as a category for lexical focus. The second measure is a modification of a procedure described by Yorkston and Beukelman (1980). In addition to the measures they employed, I also calculate syllables per content unit as an indicator of verbal efficiency.

FUNCTIONAL COMMUNICATION

Whatever gains may be achieved through either the cueing hierarchy approach or lexical focus are of little value to the patient if they do not enhance his functional communicative efficiency. I endeavor to maximize this transfer to functional situations in three ways. First, I select stimuli that are relevant to the patient's needs and interests. Second, I emphasize the development and use of internal facilitators. Much time is devoted to the levels of a cueing hierarchy that call for the patient's use of self-generated cues and to the use of search strategies in lexical focus. Third, I give the patient extensive opportunity to *communicate,* either through pragmatically based therapy approaches (see Selected References) or open conversation. It is essential that the patient have the opportunity to implement new skills and experience the communicative success that may be derived through their use.

SELECTED REFERENCES

Holland, A. Some practical considerations in aphasia rehabilitation. In M. Sullivan and M.S. Kommers (Eds.), *Rationale for Adult Aphasia Therapy.* University of Nebraska Medical Center, 1977.

LaPointe, L. Aphasia therapy: Some principles and strategies for treatment. In D.

Johns (Ed), *Clinical Management of Neurogenic Communicative Disorders*. Boston: Little, Brown and Company, 1978.

Linebaugh, C., and Lehner, L. Cueing hierarchies and word retrieval: A therapy program. In R. Brookshire (Ed.), *Clinical Aphasiology: Conference Proceedings, 1977*. Minneapolis: BRK Publishers, 1977.

Davis, G. and Wilcox, M. Incorporating parameters of natural conversation in aphasia treatment. In R. Chapey (Ed.), *Language Intervention Strategies in Adult Aphasia*. Baltimore: Williams and Wilkins, 1981.

Yorkston, K., and Beukelman, D. An analysis of connected speech samples of aphasic and normal speakers. *Journal of Speech and Hearing Disorders*, 1980, *45*:27-36.

CHAPTER FIVE

TREATMENT OF CONDUCTION APHASIA

Method of Nina N. Simmons

*"I know all these things, and I say–uh–uh–I say it and
I go on saying it–on and on, but the mainly–uh–der–worders
are very hard to say, and YOU say these to me but I just
go off into mismates–uh–mismotes– oh my goodness!"*

Hidden in this patient's somewhat vague account of his problem
is a remarkably accurate description of conduction aphasia. He has
demonstrated (1) the typically high degree of verbal fluency in the
presence of difficulty retrieving the substantive, or "main," words,
(2) the disproportionate impairment of the ability to repeat after
someone else, and (3) the frequent "mismates," or paraphasias. The
significant verbal repetition deficit accompanied by relatively intact
auditory comprehension and fluent verbal output appears to be the
hallmark of "classic" conduction aphasia. The patient's recognition
of his paraphasic errors results in hesitations and self-correction
attempts; these may seem reminiscent of apraxia of speech or Broca's
aphasia; however, the combination of fluency, preserved melody,
and variety and complexity of syntactic structures found in conduction
aphasia distinguish the disorder from nonfluent problems. The number
of paraphasic errors and the "communicative" content of speech
depend on the severity of the aphasia. The degree of reading comprehension and that of writing problems vary from patient to patient.
Overall, the salient features of conduction aphasia give the picture
of an individual who speaks with good intonation, but has trouble
retrieving words, and produces paraphasic errors which he recognizes
and tries (though often abortively) to correct.

It has been my experience that, barring serious complications,
the patient with conduction aphasia can become a functional com-
municator. Although it has been reported that patients presenting
with conduction aphasia immediately post-onset show significant,
or even complete, recovery of language function, I stumble upon
the disorder more frequently as it has evolved from a "jargon aphasia"
or Wernicke's aphasia. Because the initial presentation of such patients

45

tends to involve more severe aphasic symptoms, and probably more extensive brain lesions at onset, the "evolved" conduction aphasias exhibit more residual language deficit. Even then, I am often astounded by the ample information colorfully conveyed by a choice paraphasia which is perfectly inflected to transmit appropriate emotion, and is embedded in a context which is so revealing that the intent is perfectly clear. What is there not to understand about "Oh, no, not more Mac Donald's Damburgers?" Because of the relatively good auditory comprehension, fairly copious verbal output, and an ability to supplement speech with gestural, melodic, and facial information, these patients often function fairly well in situations that do not require single-word accuracy or specific responses. Furthermore, treatment focused appropriately results in improvements that can be documented by test-retest scores and careful charting of daily progress

PRELIMINARY TREATMENT CONSIDERATIONS

The first treatment question, of course, is whether or not to treat the patient, and if so, how often? I consider the patient with conduction aphasia to be a good treatment candidate if the usual prognostic indicators for aphasia (age, time post-onset, coexisting problems, general health, etiology, motivation, etc.) are not seriously adverse. Severity of the conduction disorder or degree of involvement in each modality will certainly influence the outcome, but does not preclude treatment; especially since conduction aphasia as a rule is considered less "severe" than those syndromes involving input as well as output deficit, such as "global" aphasia.

I prefer individual therapy as soon post-onset as possible. Maximum gains are achieved with daily therapy; however, funding, scheduling options, transportation problems, or staff shortages often preclude such intensive scheduling. My patients tolerate and profit from hour-long sessions when they are geared to promote success and this keeps the patient functioning at a maximum level without allowing failure. Fatigue and frustration seem to surge when a session falls short of this goal.

Education and Counseling

A major issue that must be addressed early on is counseling and educating the patient and family. I begin this in the first session and continue throughout treatment:

1. A discussion of general characteristics of brain damage—such as fatigability, interference effects, and noise build-up—is initiated immediately. The family is introduced to family groups, or a "Stroke Club," to gain support, and given access to a lending library for additional information. The nature of the discussion varies from family to family, often resulting in ongoing counseling and information exchange.

2. As soon as specific information is gleaned from testing, I discuss the nature of the disorder with the family—what is wrong *and* what is right with the patient. I attempt to find out their goals and expectations, and explain my goals and expectations.

3. I try to learn how the family interacts with the patient and what strategies they use that promote or hinder communication. We talk about ways to facilitate communication, such as recognizing when to allow the patient more time to elaborate, or when to stop and ask for clarification, when to overlook paraphasic "errors," and when to acknowledge them.

4. I discuss test results, the nature of conduction aphasia, and rationale of treatment with the patient (without the family present). I consider it important that the patient be included in goal setting and planning from the outset.

GENERAL GOALS AND PRINCIPLES

While each type of aphasia differs in specific behaviors, there are a number of general goals and principles. The overall goals include:

1. Defining the behaviors with which the patient has trouble, finding a level at which he can perform the behaviors successfully, and practicing at this level in an effort to improve performance.

2. Providing ways in which responses are facilitated.

3. Helping the patient develop compensatory strategies aimed at increasing the success of communication.

These goals, and the general principles of stimulation therapy for aphasia (Brookshire, 1978), form a foundation upon which my therapy approach is built. Given an understanding of the general principles of aphasia treatment, specific problems of conduction aphasia can be addressed. Approaching treatment by categorizing aphasias by no means precludes assessment of individual strengths and weaknesses and targeting individual behaviors. Applying the label of "conduction aphasia" merely lights the stage whereupon one must look at, listen to, and evaluate the individual player.

STRUCTURE OF THE THERAPY SESSION

The treatment session follows a general framework involving an initial period of conversation to find out "What's been happenin'!" The patient's mood, energy level, and relevant news can be important determinants of the direction of the session and the clinician's behavior. From here, we move into easy warm-up activities, slowly increase the difficulty of activities, and finally ease off into relatively simple "cool-down" activities. I attempt to end each session on a successful note, discussing performance and pointing out areas of improvement and those areas needing more work.

Basic to this format is an understanding of the task hierarchy concept. This is a method of organizing and introducing therapy tasks which slowly increase in difficulty level by small steps until I have faded control, and the patient has increased his level of performance. Therapy activities begin where the patient can function; they evolve out of an understanding of what makes a response easier or more difficult, and they evolve out of an understanding of the many variables affecting the patient's performance (Darley, 1976). There are no "universal" hierarchies applicable to all conduction aphasias. Each plan must result from the individual patient's behavior. Furthermore, no hierarchy is immutable. Alas, one must accept the challenge of entering a session with a beautifully organized continuum of activities only to be diverted onto a totally different track, following the patient's lead.

I find the easiest way to know what is going on in the session, when to diverge and when to trudge forward, is to score each response using PICA scores *(Porch Index of Communicative Ability)*, and organize activities on a score sheet. I complete 10 trials on each task for ease in computing averages. Also a base-10 format (La Pointe, 1977) is helpful in recording baseline performance, progress over time, and information on efficacy of techniques. To arrive at each task, I determine the stimulus modality, the response modality, the number of items in the field, the stimulus-response interval, the rate and manner of stimulus presentation, the number and sequence of trials, and the type of cues or prompts to be used. The tasks can be hypothetically ordered from easy to difficult (for *each* patient), as in Table 1. I must admit that I no longer routinely write out a complete hierarchy prior to treatment. It seems that after this ordeal has been experienced many times, the concepts become indelibly traced on the appropriate brain cells, allowing the experienced clinician to approach treatment sessions with a general plan that can be thoughtfully varied and manipulated to produce desired responses. The score sheet, then, documents the results and represents the task continuum, which evolved from patient behavior.

I attempt to provide feedback that is relevant, specific, and as "positive" as possible. In other words, instead of saying, "Oh, no—that's wrong," I might say, "You were close—watch that last syllable—it's libra*ry*." Better yet, appropriate tasks and stimuli should not produce error responses; errors suggest a need to alter the requirements of the activity or to slip in "preventative" cues. Reinforcement for correct responses should facilitate a relaxed atmosphere. Although I realize the need to avoid undue distraction, I abhor the

TABLE 1   Portion of a Therapy Task Continuum Designed for a Specific Patient

Task	Stimulus	Response	S-R Interval	Rate/Manner/Items
1. Say common 1-syllable nouns	Auditory (noun) Visual (writ.noun)	Verbal	Immediate, written noun present	Normal 10 nouns
2. Say common 1-syllable nouns	Auditory (noun) Visual (writ. noun)	Verbal	2 sec. delay, written noun removed	Normal Same nouns
3. Repeat nouns	Auditory (noun) (fade visual)	Verbal	Immediate	Normal Same nouns
4. TASKS 1-3 with common 1-syllable verbs				
5. Say sentences (You (verb) a (noun)	Auditory (sent.) Visual (writ. sent.)	Verbal Gestural (point as read word)	Immediate written sent. present	Slow, pauses same nouns and verbs
6. Say sentences	Auditory (sent.) Visual (writ. sent.)	Verbal Gestural	2 sec. delay written sent. removed	Slow, pauses Same nouns
7. Repeat sentences	Auditory (fade visual)	Verbal	Immediate	Slow, pauses Same nouns
8. Complete a spoken & written sentence (You (verb) a __)	Auditory (incomp. sent.) Visual (writ. incomp. sent.)	Verbal (noun)	Immediate	Stress verb, Same nouns and verbs

repetitious, hollow, or saccharine "goooods" which seem to echo through aphasia clinics. I would much prefer a lively, albeit off-color, "Hey, you got that sucker!" While obviously the timbre of the session should suit the personalities of those involved, I find that humor and a variety of comments are consistently appreciated.

TARGETING THE PROBLEM

The next step is to pinpoint the specific behaviors that are most frequently targeted in conduction aphasia.

Auditory Comprehension

While intact auditory comprehension is considered, by definition, a characteristic of conduction aphasia, patients often thoughtlessly refuse to fit into our tidy definitions. It is not unusual to find patients who broadly adhere to the conduction aphasia profile, but *do* have involvement of the auditory channel. Such is the case as a "jargon aphasia" begins to improve in the direction of conduction aphasia. When auditory deficits exist, I include this area in therapy. I employ traditional "point to" and direction-following task continuums in which sentence or word length, syntactic complexity, rate of speech, field, stimulus-response interval, redundancy, etc. are systematically manipulated to build responsivity. I also encourage the patient to develop listening tactics (such as asking for repeats, simplification, or pauses).

Verbal Repetition

Unlike treatment of other aphasias, therapy of conduction aphasia does not include verbal imitation as a powerful technique in deblocking access to spoken words. Because repetition is a primary deficit, it becomes a target of treatment rather than an approach to treatment. Although proficiency in repeating after other people is not a particularly useful skill, it seems that as verbal repetition improves, other behaviors (such as self-correcting and word retrieval) follow suit. On occasion I have found verbal repetition deficits do not respond to treatment; in these cases, attention is obviously redirected to more functional areas.

Focusing therapy on verbal imitation involves (1) determining the level at which repetition begins to deteriorate, (2) determining the influences of variables such as word length, frequency of occurrence, phonemic complexity, and part of speech, and (3) determining what facilitates the patient's verbal repetition. For instance, despite problems in reading aloud, many patients are significantly facilitated on repeating a spoken word when the written word is provided. With an understanding of those variables that allow easy imitation, I initiate treatment across a continuum of activities with sufficient successful practice at each level to indicate a need to move on. Steps can be made easier or harder by varying the length of the words or phrases, speaking the word in unison with the patient, or enforcing delays (and even "filled" delays) between the spoken word and the patient's response, providing "facial" or phonemic cues, varying syntactic or grammatic complexity, and so forth.

Word Retrieval

Since "anomia" is characteristic of these patients, targeting word retrieval is useful. I consider it ineffectual to simply direct a patient to say the names of things over and over. In fact, word drills (even when prompts or facilitators are used) are of little value if there is no effort to internalize strategies for accessing vocabulary and improving the level of performance. Activities that provide practice of word retrieval under facilitory conditions (using word associations, high imagery pictures, written cues, gestural cues) and systematically increase the demand for "independent" word finding should improve the process of retrieving words. An infinite variety of tasks are suitable for this sort of thing; a few based on word association cues are listed in Table 2. An interesting observation is that phonemic cues (saying the initial sound or syllable) are far less powerful cues for these patients than they are with the "anterior" aphasias. Many times I have cleverly slipped in an initial sound cue only to elicit a paraphasic error with the correct initial sound! Actually, over the course of treatment, and as repetition and word retrieval improve, the use of phonemic cues becomes more appropriate. (I sometimes wonder if this is because, inadvertently, I have trained the patient to use the cue instead of using the cue to train the patient!)

While incorporating visual, written, gestural and/or auditory cues into word retrieval practice, I assist the patient in developing successful strategies and self-cueing techniques. If clinician-provided word associations ("drive a _____") or gestures (pantomime driving) facilitate word recall, the patient can be directed to use these himself.

TABLE 2   A Sample of Verbal Word Retrieval Tasks of Varying Word Association Strength

Task	Example
1. Paired associates	"Shoes and ____."
2. Complete a spoken sentence with the written word provided	"You drive a ____." (show written word CAR)
3. Complete a spoken sentence with a picture provided	"You drive a ____." (show picture of car)
4. Complete a spoken sentence	"You drive a ____."
5. Answer a structured question	"What do you *drive?*"
6. Answer a question	"You drive this. What do you call it?"
7. Answer a low-association question	"What do you call this?" (show picture of car)

For instance, the patient who recognizes a paraphasic error, and compounds the error on repeated self-correction attempts, might redirect his efforts at finding an associated word (what you *do* with it) or using a gesture to self-cue. I might note that even if these cues do not assist in retrieving the specific word, they serve the additional purpose of communicating the intent in the absence of a productive self-correcting system.

Sentence Structure

Although I encourage circumlocutory or "divergent" strategies to convey ideas successfully, I also devise a segment of treatment aimed at structured, specific verbal responses at the sentence level. The patient with conduction aphasia uses a variety of grammatic and syntactic structures, and lots of words, but, in the barrage of fluent speech, the good is lost in the bad. For this reason, I concentrate on verbalizing specific sentence structures (such as: The *noun* is *verb*ing), using whatever variables assist with production. For instance, the patient might read each word of a sentence, or form a sentence given a noun, with the goal of *controlling* fluency. Judicious use of pauses and slow rate inhibit the tendency to launch furiously into verbiage. Instead of using "stop strategies" requiring exclamations of "slow down," "think," or other equally annoying reminders, I prefer to pace the activity or use gestural accompaniment. Pointing to each word as it is spoken, or using a pacing board to slow the rate, allows processing pauses and focuses attention. When the patient successfully formulates structured sentences, the stop strategies can be incorporated into picture description, answering questions, and more open-ended tasks. During these activities, I attempt to build an awareness that vague responses can be as noncommunicative as errors; however, it is important that the individual patient is ready for this type of approach. It would be unwise to "inhibit" fluency and circumlocutory strategies without a foundation of retrieval potential.

Reading and Writing

Treating of the patient with conduction aphasia covers all areas of deficit, including reading and writing. These areas are treated within the structure of language therapy; therefore, stimulus items used on reading comprehension tasks might be carried over into verbal and writing activities to "prime" the system for responses later on in the session. Short words and phrases from repetition and word retrieval work might be incorporated into copying and writing tasks to minimize the need for "shifting." My overall approach to reading and writing reflects the same orientation and is incorporated into the treatment of auditory-verbal channels; therefore, further discussion is unnecesary.

Functional Communication

Since the goal of treatment is to have the patient communicating outside of the structure and support of therapy, I direct some attention to the natural conversation setting. PACE therapy (Wilcox and Davis, 1981) can meet this need for the patient with conduction aphasia. The goal of functional communication activities might be to encourage use of channels in addition to verbal ones, to point out nonproductive self-correct behavior, to reinforce successful communication strategies, to desensitize the patient to listener responses (failure to understand, etc.), to reinforce use of facial expressions, and so on.

FACILITORY CHANNELS

Visual Cues

In spite of impairment in reading comprehension or oral reading, the visual channel (graphic cues) often proves helpful in strengthening access to desired responses. Initially providing written cues during verbal language tasks, then slowly fading the written cues, seems to help. Perhaps shifting some responsibility for accessing words to another system and practicing at this level alters response patterns somehow. (It has been suggested that in some conduction aphasias, sparing of the superior longitudinal fasciculus allows visual information to be transmittted anteriorly while auditory information is blocked.) At any rate, for patients with no significant visual involvement, I have used graphic cues at all levels of treatment.

Gestural Cues

Gesture has proven a very useful channel with conduction aphasia patients. Although these patients often exhibit "limb apraxias" and may not spontaneously use symbolic or creative gestures, this modality can be strengthened and incorporated into treatment to facilitate word recall. The best approach I have found involves building fast and accurate recognition and production of symbolic gesture (such as Amerind signs) by structuring tasks around pictures of sign production, written word and sentence cues, producing the sign in response to spoken or written words, phrases, or questions, and finally including the sign in verbal expressive tasks. Initial practice of gestures without encouraging simultaneous verbal responses often reduces useless "empty" verbiage. When used to facilitate verbal output, gestures seem to help direct attention to the specific idea to be communicated.

Rhythm and Song

I have not found Melodic Intonation Therapy or prosodic cueing to be successful approaches in improving the verbal expression of the patient with conduction aphasia.

RESULTS

No single chapter can possibly encapsulate every aspect of treatment. In writing this chapter, I began to think there were as many different approaches to conduction aphasia as there were conduction aphasic patients. Of course, I do many things with other types of patients (extensive auditory work with Wernicke's, syntax programs with Broca's, using stress and rhythm with apraxia of speech) that I do not do with conduction patients, and it occurred to me that the purpose of this chapter is simply to narrow the "field" of therapy choices a bit without providing the proverbial "cookbook." By carefully applying knowledge of prognostic variables, principles of aphasia treatment, learning theory, and relevant research, I have achieved good results with the approaches described. Conduction aphasic patients properly diagnosed and selected for treatment may not become "perfect," but they generally get better; as the patient quoted at the beginning of the chapter stated after months of therapy: "Now I can really say everything. Remember when I used to mess up a lot. Boy! Now I never make tistakes!"

SELECTED REFERENCES

Brookshire, R. *An Introduction to Aphasia.* Minneapolis: BRK Publishers, 1978.

Darley, F. Maximizing input to the aphasic patient. In R. Brookshire (Ed.), *Clinical Aphasiology Conference Proceedings, 1976.* Minneapolis: BRK Publishers, 1976.

Davis, G., and Wilcox, M. Natural conversation in aphasia treatment. In R. Chapey (Ed.), *Language Intervention Strategies in Adult Aphasia.* Baltimore: Williams and Wilkins, 1981.

LaPointe, L. Base-10 programmed stimulation: Task specification, scoring, and plotting performance in aphasia therapy. *Journal of Speech and Hearing Disorders,* 1977, 42:90.

CHAPTER SIX

TREATMENT OF RIGHT HEMISPHERE COMMUNICATION DISORDERS

Method of Penelope Starratt Myers

Providing treatment for the general communication deficits associated with unilaterial right cerebral hemisphere (RH) damage is a relatively new development. Until very recently, speech pathologists working with this population restricted their treatment to motor speech disorders, occasionally including work on reading and writing deficits. Many professionals, however, have had the intuitive feeling that their RH patients suffered from other more subtle, but no less critical, communication impairments. But only in the last five years or so have research data from split-brain, brain-damaged, and normal subjects begun to replace intuition, so that systematic, data-based judgment can be applied in providing treatment.

Because this area of study is still in its infancy, several cautionary notes should precede a discussion of treatment:

1. The operations of the intact RH are not as clearly understood, or as well defined, as are those of the left hemisphere (LH).

2. Not all RH patients manifest the symptoms to be described herein. Symptoms vary with site and size of lesion, with degree of handedness and hemispheric dominance, and in some cases with the educational and professional background of the patient. In addition, localization studies on RH communication disorders are almost nonexistent.

3. Adequate diagnostic tools do not exist in published form. Standard aphasia tests can and should be used, but with caution. RH communication deficits do not fall on a continuum of aphasia or aphasia-like behaviors. Although it is true that RH patients make errors on these tests due to specific language impairments, many of their other deficits cannot be accounted for in an aphasia battery. Errors by RH patients on aphasia tests are often the result of impaired visual perceptual skills rather than as a language deficit. Scoring systems are usually not designed to account for problems specific to RH damage. Finally, the stimuli in most aphasia batteries are not

57

sophisticated or open-ended enough to demonstrate potential RH disorders. Thus, one may end with a depressed score for the wrong reasons, or an elevated score because the test was not designed to assess the types of communication deficits that may exist despite adequate linguistic skills. As long as these precautions are observed, aphasia tests can and should be used—with other formal and informal tests that include less concrete and more sophisticated communication demands. Aphasia tests are useful in determining whether or not the patient has some specific linguistic deficits, and in providing an opportunity to note the patient's communicative behavior during testing, regardless of the adequacy of the scoring system.

What follows, then, is a description of RH disorders and suggestions for treatment. Although the chapter is current now, new information from research and clinical experience will ensure that it is not written in stone.

RH communication disorders can be divided into three broad categories that are interrelated—each can have an impact on the other two. The categories are: (1) visuo-spatial deficits, which include problems resulting from left-side neglect and very basic perceptual discrimination impairments; (2) linguistic processing deficits, which include specific language problems; and (3) higher order perceptual and cognitive deficits, which include those impairments that result in general communicative inefficiency. This last category covers those problems that are often characterized as inappropriate, literal, irrelevant, and sometimes bizarre communicative behavior. As will be seen in Category III, many of these deficits stem directly and indirectly from disorders in the first two categories. Each of these three categories and the treatment procedures specific to them will be discussed separately below.

CATEGORY I: VISUO-SPATIAL DEFICITS

Visuo-spatial deficits associated with RH damage include: (1) impaired visual discrimination, (2) impaired short-term visual memory, (3) impaired scanning and tracking, (4) impaired facial recognition (prosopagnosia), (5) impaired topological and geographic orientation, (6) impaired body-schema (anosagnosia), (7) constructional apraxia, (8) dressing apraxia, and (9) left-sided neglect. Most of these impairments have a direct impact on regaining independence in self-care activities. Many of them have an impact on visually based communication skills. Prosopagnosia, for example, can make it difficult for the patient to recognize family members or to distinguish the characters in a television drama. Constructional apraxia may impair grapheme production. Deficits in scanning and tracking will impede reading. Left-sided neglect may affect all of these skills. Theories about the cause of neglect abound, but regardless of the cause, it is generally accepted that severe neglect results in a loss of concept— not only for the left side of the body, but for the entire left half of space. Neglect is often accompanied by denial of the affected limbs and, in some patients, by denial of illness. It can severely impair reading. Unlike hemianopsia, which prevents the patient from seeing a portion of the page, neglect inhibits the patient's ability to conceive of, and therefore to look at, the left side of space, whether a printed page or the scene in front of him.

The following treatment strategies are geared toward improving the perceptual skills necessary to reading and writing. Reading comprehension and graphic expression deficits will be covered in Category II.

I take three steps before providing treatment. First, I distinguish between reading and writing deficits that are perceptual and those that are linguistic. Second, I make sure that the patient is aware of his problems. This is a necessary step when providing any type of communication therapy to the RH patient, who is notable for a lack of motivation in the rehabilitation process. This attitude can sometimes be traced to denial of illness, but in the area of communication it is often based simply on lack of awareness and misinformation. Family and staff members, relieved that the patient does not have aphasia, convince him that he should have no communication problems whatsoever. Some patients fear that the problems they are experiencing may be linked to more extensive brain damage, or to psychological disturbance. In other patients, poor self-monitoring can be confused with true denial. I have found that most patients are relieved to admit to communication disorders when they trust the therapist, when they learn that treatment exists, and when they realize that their problems are neither unusual nor unexpected.

Third, if the patient is also undergoing occupational therapy, I consult that therapist before embarking on a treatment program for the visual-perceptual deficits associated with reading and writing. Occupational therapists are specifically trained to work on visual-perceptual disorders; duplication of their efforts by the speech-language pathologist is a waste of valuable treatment time. In addition, the occupational therapist should be able to provide the speech clinician with useful test data, plus information about the existence and severity of left-sided neglect.

Reading Tasks

Task 1: Right-Left Matching
a. Task Explanation:

The goal of this task is to heighten awareness of the left side of the page. The patient is required to match a single stimuli on the right with one of several on the left.

b. Stimuli:

Begin with simple familiar geometric shapes and move to upper and lower case letters. At the lowest level, stimuli should be three-dimensional to allow tactile as well as visual stimulation. Later, they should be printed.

c. Program Levels:

(1) Match forms, then letters, by moving the one on the right next to its match on the left. Eventually have the patient match them by drawing a connecting line.

(2) Gradually increase the number of foils and move stimuli on the left further away from the center.

(3) Fade tactile cues—use printed letters and, eventually, simple words.

Task 2: Scanning
a. Task Explanation:

The patient is required to scan a horizontal line of letters circling a target letter.

b. Stimuli:

Begin with widely spaced large letters, gradually decreasing their size and the amount of space between them.

c. Program Levels:

At first, arrange letters vertically to the patient's right and later use a horizontal arrangement while lengthening the line on both sides of the center point.

Task 3: Visual Sequential Memory
a. Task Explanation:

This task is designed to improve short-term visual memory and sequencing skills as well as to heighten left-sided awareness. The patient observes a series of stimuli arranged horizontally for a brief period of time and duplicates the arrangement without looking at the model.

b. Stimuli:

Pictured geometric shapes on small cards. Avoid left hemisphere involvement by omitting letters or objects which the patient can name, unless this is preferred as an initial step.

c. Program Levels:

(1) Begin with as few as two and move up to as many as five shapes.

(2) Allow as many repetitions as necessary, gradually fading them before adding more stimuli.

(3) Gradually decrease viewing time.

(4) Allow patient to copy model before moving to reproduction from memory.

Task 4: Reading Sentences Aloud

a. Task Explanation:

The goal of this task is accurate oral reading, not reading comprehension.

b. Stimuli:

Begin with simple active declarative sentences, gradually increasing length and linguistic complexity.

c. Cues:

Red margin marker on the left.

Verbal cue directing patient to look to the left.

Verbal self-cue by patient.

Patient points to each word with his finger.

d. Program Levels:

(1) Begin with large print and simple sentences, gradually moving to smaller, more closely spaced print and more complex sentences.

(2) Fade cues and re-introduce them as necessary, as sentences and print become more difficult to read.

(3) If patient cannot manage without verbal self-cue or margin marker, encourage him to continue their use in all reading.

Task 5: Reading Paragraphs

Follow the steps and procedures in task 4, "Reading Sentences." Programs from paragraphs printed in large type to newspaper or other columned material to material that is printed across a page. Make use of the patient's own reading material in therapy.

Writing Tasks

Among the grapheme production deficits that may occur with RH damage are perseveration and/or omission of strokes, graphemes, syllables, punctuation marks such as commas and periods, and capital letters. Sentences tend to slant upward and to be produced without regard to margins. Words and letters are often poorly spaced. Constructional apraxia may contribute to graphic problems. I test the patient for this disorder by having him copy a clock face, flower, cross, and square. If he omits the left side, or detail on the left, or places extraneous detail on the right, I begin treatment with Tasks 1 and 2. If not, I proceed to Tasks 3 and 4.

Task 1: Drawing
a. Task Explanation:
   Patient is required to draw familiar forms and objects.
b. Stimuli:
   Symmetrical geometric shapes and familiar figures.
c. Program levels:
   Progress from tracing to copying to reproducing from memory to spontaneous production, using a felt-tip pen.

Task 2: Simple Word Production
   Follow procedures outlined in Task 1.

Task 3: Simple Sentences
a. Task Explanation:
   Patient is required to copy simple sentences.
b. Stimuli:
   See Task 5, under Reading Tasks.
c. Program Levels:
   Use the same cueing hierarchy described in reading sentences aloud (Task 5). Begin with print and move to script. Fade all but self-generated cues. Use lined paper at first.

Task 4: Spontaneous Written Expression
a. Task Explanation:
   Picture description.
b. Stimuli:
   Simple action pictures moving to more complex ones.
c. Program Levels:
   (1) Provide patient with a written sentence describing a picture in a sentence completion task.
   (2) Spontaneous simple active declarative sentences.
   (3) Complex picture description requiring a simple paragraph or more complex and lengthy sentence.
   (4) See cueing hierarchy in Task 5, under Reading.

CATEGORY II: LINGUISTIC DEFICITS

Although it is a mistake to characterize RH communication impairment as aphasia, standard aphasia testing will often reveal some specific linguistic disorders. Generally, deficits found in aphasia testing will be receptive rather than expressive in nature. Depressed scores on simple expressive tasks such as confrontation naming are often due to delayed responses rather than to errors in naming per se. The complex visual array of the test stimuli can contribute to visual-perceptual problems during testing. Low verbal fluency scores associated with RH damage are probably less the result of naming or categorization problems than of problems in the control of available linguistic information. Aberrations in other, higher-order expressive tasks such as picture descriptions are usually the result of the cognitive and experiential deficits explored in Category III, rather than a language impairment.

Auditory comprehension errors appear to be a function of the level of linguistic complexity and degree of embedding, rather than a function of length. Short-term auditory memory tasks such as digit recall and following three- or four-stage commands rarely present problems. On the other hand, reading comprehension impairments in many cases are a function of length as well as level of complexity. This is perhaps because visual-perceptual problems interfere with and disrupt the efficient comprehension of visual symbols.

These receptive language deficits and any other specific linguistic disorders found in RH patients should, I believe, be treated in the same manner as any other language deficit. The general stimulation techniques used in aphasia therapy (breaking complex tasks into small steps, then progressing logically through increasingly more demanding stages) should be very effective with RH patients. This technique relies on the kind of processing in which the LH is thought to predominate.

CATEGORY III: HIGHER ORDER COMMUNICATION DEFICITS

In addition to the specific linguistic and perceptual disorders just described, RH patients demonstrate a range of deficits on so-phisticated communication tasks. These deficits are most apparent when the patient is engaged in an involved conversation—when asked to describe a pictured situation, explain a joke, tell a story, or respond to open-ended questions. The less concrete the task requirements, the more likely the patient is to demonstrate the following types of problems: (1) difficulty in organizing information in an efficient, meaningful way; (2) a tendency to produce impulsive, poorly thought-out answers that are rife with tangential and related, but unnecessary, detail; (3) difficulty in distinguishing between what is important and what is not; (4) problems in assimilating and using contextual cues; (5) a tendency to lend a literal interpretation to figurative language; (6) a tendency to overpersonalize external events; and (7) a reduced sensitivity to the communicative situation and the pragmatic aspects of communication.

In order to provide effective treatment for these "extralinguistic" deficits, I think it is necessary to explore the common threads weaving them together. Research with split-brain and normal subjects has postulated—and, indeed, the common wisdom now accepts—that the two hemispheres have differing processing styles. The LH is thought to predominate in linear analytic thinking, decoding by feature analysis. The RH is thought to predominate in the synthesis and simultaneous integration of parts into wholes, and to reason by a nonlinear mode of association (see Selected References). The effects of an impairment in RH processing can be demonstrated on both a perceptual and a higher cognitive level. For example, RH patients perform very poorly on visual integration tasks in which they must label a pictured object that has been broken apart into its component pieces, even when they can match the picture to one of four choices. On a higher level, this deficit has been found to impair their ability to extract critical bits of information, see the relationships among them, and draw inferences based on those relationships. Many RH patients thus find it difficult to weigh and interpret what they see. Descriptions of pictured events and situations become a rather random list of featured items, rather than an explanation of events.

Most of the disorders in this section can be traced to the impaired perception of experience itself—perception not only at its most basic level of discrimination and identification, but on a higher cognitive plane as well. Perception on this higher level is that unique ability in man which makes him more than a sensory recorder, which enables him to discriminate and interpret at the same time, and which helps him relate the fragments of experience into a personal whole. The patient's altered perception of experience results in a reduced ability to utilize context in the search for meaning. It makes it difficult for him to determine the communicative requirements of a given situation—to grasp his listener's needs, his level of responsiveness, and to understand the illocutionary force of a message. In addition, deficits in the association of and control over internal information impair his ability to direct, channel, and organize verbal expression. He thus tends to itemize rather than explain, and to include irrelevant detail as he drifts off into a tangential area.

I base treatment for these disorders on tasks that do the following: (1) encourage the use of contextual cues and contextually conveyed meaning, (2) require the patient to make verbal and visual associations,

(3) encourage him to integrate what he sees and hears and to interpret rather than itemize, and (4) require him to demonstrate an understanding of the pragmatic rules of conversation—from turn-taking to understanding what is meant from what is said. In general, low-level tasks have highly specific convergent response requirements, while higher order tasks are more divergent and open-ended in nature.

Sample Communication Tasks

Task 1: Integrating Contextual Cues—Visual Presentation
a. Task Explanation:
>   The patient is required to utilize contextual cues in explaining and interpreting a pictured scene. This is not a picture *description* task.
b. Stimuli:
>   Pictured scenes ranging from simple actor-action pictures to more complex situations. The complexity of the higher level stimuli should depend not on the number of elements, but on subtle interactions and relationships between elements. At this level, the task should require the patient to reach conclusions through inferential reasoning.
c. Program Levels:
>   (1) Patient labels items in picture.
>   (2) Patient explains actions and events. In early stages, the patient may need prompting through the use of "wh" questions. These cues should eventually be faded so that the patient provides an adequate interpretation on his own.

Task 2: Integrating Contextual Cues—Auditory Presentation
a. Task Explanation:
>   The patient reads, or is read, a brief story and must answer questions that demonstrate knowledge not only of what took place in the story, but of why it took place.
b. Stimuli:
>   Stories ranging from simple action stories in which events are logical and predictable (i.e., boy falls down, runs to mother, gets Band-aid) to ones in which the story line is somewhat unpredictable, and in which some of the information is inferred, rather than stated directly.
c. Program Levels:
>   (1) Lowest level—patient must answer questions about the action, i.e., "What," "Where," "When" questions.
>   (2) Highest level—patient must answer not only "what" but

"why" questions, i.e., generate conclusions based on the context of the events. Conclusions must be based on the events in the story, not on the personal history of the patient.

Task 3: Divergent Questions

a. Task Explanation:

This task or series of tasks is directed at the pragmatic aspects of communication. Open-ended questions are embedded in conversation, and the patient's ability to follow conversational rules and to stay on the topic are monitored.

b. Stimuli:

Preprogrammed open-ended or divergent questions related to personal or current events.

c. Program Levels:

Both turn-taking and the patient's ability to stay on the topic are monitored by the clinician through whatever means the clinician deems appropriate, e.g., raising his/her hand when patient digresses. Use of video or audio tapes is helpful. Eventually, external cues are faded as patient begins to monitor himself.

Task 4: Tell a Story

a. Task Explanation:

The patient is asked to tell a brief story based on a pictured stimulus. The story is judged for the degree to which it is coherent and complete.

b. Stimuli:

Picture cards ranging from simple sequential cards to ones that are emotionally evocative.

c. Program Levels:

See stimuli—the patient should be required to move from stories that follow a simple chronological sequence to ones that interpret and explain emotions expressed in the pictured stimulus.

SELECTED REFERENCES

Adamovich, B., and Brooks, R., A diagnostic protocol to assess the communication deficits of patients with right hemisphere damage. In R. Brookshire (Ed.), *Clinical Aphasiology: Conference Proceedings,* Minneapolis: BRK Publishers, 1981.

Gardner, H . *The Shattered Mind.* New York: Vintage Books, 1974

Gazzaniga, M. *The Bisected Brain.* New York: Appleton-Century-Crofts, 1970.

Myers, P. Profiles of communication deficits in patients with right cerebral hemisphere damage; Implications for diagnosis and treatment. In R. Brookshire (Ed.), *Clinical Aphasiology: Conference Proceedings*. Minneapolis: BRK Publishers, 1979.

Myers, P. Treatment of right hemisphere patients, panel discussion. In R. Brookshire (Ed.), *Clinical Aphasiology: Conference Proceedings*. Minneapolis: BRK Publishers, 1981

CHAPTER SEVEN

TREATMENT OF ALEXIA WITH AGRAPHIA

Method of Wanda G. Webb

The treatment procedures for the acquired reading and writing deficits in adults cannot be written out on a prescription pad and meted out to every client. Each individual brings to the session his or her own premorbid literacy history, method of attacking "academically oriented" assignments, and personal interests and motivation regarding reading and writing. The clinician must become informed about these, if possible, and must be creative and flexible in the approach to establishing the desired goals. The strategies and order of presentation of the methods and materials herein described, therefore, must be considered only suggestions and guidelines. No two clients will need the same program or materials for reading and writing tasks.

The majority of the methodologies and tasks in this chapter have been learned from other clinicians who have shared ideas with their colleagues through the literature. The therapy procedures are given according to personally defined severity levels. These severity levels are operationally defined according to my clinical standards. This rating follows diagnostic testing and is not based on a particular test's standard, but rather on observed overall performance. In writing about these procedures, it is presumed that the client also has other language deficits that are being treated simultaneously, and that the procedures will have to be modified according to the limitations imposed by these deficits.

STIMULUS DESIGN

Several criteria should be kept in mind when purchasing or creating stimulus materials to use in the client's program for reading and writing. One of the most important is that the stimuli should be as interesting and salient as possible. These two features provide motivation and facilitate performance. Other features of words, phrases, or sentences that research has shown may contribute to the ease with which they are read or written are: (1) length, (2) degree of abstraction, (3) imagery value (how easily they may be visualized in the "mind's eye"), (4) grammatical complexity, (5) frequency of occurrence in the language, and (6) familiarity to the user.

69

THE CLIENT WITH A SEVERE DEFICIT

The individual with a severe deficit is one who is able to indicate comprehension of very few single words, does not read text, and is unable to write anything beyond his/her name and perhaps some overlearned material such as serial numbers. There is usually poor letter recognition as well. This poor performance in reading is present whether the task is silent or oral reading.

I believe the immediate goal with this client is the use of very functional reading recognition skills and simple functional writing skill. I place emphasis on recognition and comprehension of "environmental notices," such as restroom signs, traffic signs, store names, phone numbers for emergency use, and labels on foods and other needed items. Writing goals should include name and address, the alphabet in sequence (this may not be a reasonable goal for some), ability to take down numbers from dictation, and ability to copy accurately so that checks may be written.

The client may need to be started on word-to-word matching tasks in which the visual similarity of the words is gradually increased. Word domino games are often enjoyable ways to accomplish this. The criteria should be 100 percent accuracy with rapid performance. Along with this, or following this, I may ask clients to match words to a verbal-combined-with-a-picture stimulus. These may be pictures of everyday objects, which should have labels, such as restroom doors, stop signs, storefront names, and business names (hospital, bank, school). For clients who have little difficulty with those, I move on to matching words to object pictures, such as chair, shoe, radio, suitcase, refrigerator, pen, etc. I let the person hear and see the correct word matched with the correct item as often as needed to stimulate recognition and comprehension. The audio card readers are excellent for this repeated stimulation.

Since there is often an accompanying hemiplegia in these cases, it is frequently necessary to have the nondominant hand used for writing. Copying tasks using geometric figures, and then moving to the alphabet in sequence, are useful to begin the therapy for the agraphia. As soon as copying is at least 75 percent accurate, the client should begin writing his/her name, address, and phone number. Copying the stimulus, covering it, then writing from memory, rechecking, correcting, and writing again from memory is a sequence that is usually beneficial. This sequence enables clients to practice independently if they are good at visual monitoring.

THE CLIENT WITH A MODERATELY SEVERE DEFICIT

A moderately severe deficit is operationally defined as inability to read beyond the single word and simple phrase level. Writing is adequate but slow for simple, concrete single words or simple phrases. Word-to-word association tasks using concrete nouns matched with less frequent descriptor or associated nouns and verbs (example: "pillow" with "soft" or "rest") help begin moving the client toward recognition of less frequent, more abstract words. Phrase-to-picture matching helps those who do not easily comprehend the phrases, even though they can be read word by word. The choices may be gradually made more similar so that the phrases may eventually differ by only one word.

I teach the meaning of useful abstract verbs such as "put," "give," "lay," and "turn" early so that written directions may be followed. Locatives such as "in," "on," "under," "to the left," must also be taught early.

Often, the person will choose to read aloud, and this may be very helpful to the clinician. The types of errors made can be categorized as to visual, semantic, or auditory confusions. Other types of errors may be more difficult to define. My reading the short phrases aloud in unison with the client may help to cue the perception and recognition of words and help make the reading more fluent. After reading aloud in unison, the client should be asked to read aloud alone, then to read silently, and be given a chance to demonstrate comprehension. This system forces one to go slowly and try to read each word.

The client who is beginning to be able to follow written directions may also begin to read very short and very simple stories (two to three sentences). Sentences that explain pictures are best since the person will get clues from the picture as well. As reading improves, the pictures may be withdrawn and the complexity of the sentences increased.

These clients should be simultaneously working on writing with the reading material. Copying again can be used and accuracy should be emphasized. They may be asked to copy the phrases they are reading as well as the short stories. They may begin to copy the alphabet and quickly move to writing it from memory. For some, writing the letter in the air with large movements helps reinforce the desired association. Letters may then be randomly dictated, as may short simple words. Chaining may be used to help learn to write difficult words. Chaining involves progressively omitting letters from the word until they are spelling the word on their own (matches; matche _ ; match __ ; matc ___ ; mat ____ ; ma _____ ; m _____ ; _____).

Last, the client should be building a written vocabulary of functional nouns and verbs and gradually adding the locatives, adjectives, and small grammatical words to write simple sentences.

THE CLIENT WITH A MODERATE DEFICIT

Moderate deficit is operationally defined as the inability to read at a higher instructional level (i.e., 75 percent comprehension) than third or fourth grade reading material. In writing, there is obvious difficulty with spelling. Sentences are attempted, but there are many grammatical errors.

These clients may be able to use phonetic cues in reading and, therefore, a trial at relearning sound-symbol association is worthwhile. They should be able to tell me if any phonics were previously learned. If there is no memory of attempting phonics, it may not be useful to try. If they, however, think "sounding out" may have been learned previously, or if there is willingness to try to learn some of the more frequent consonants, this might be helpful. Common word analysis and synthesis skills as are taught in normal reading work at the elementary level may also be helpful for reading and writing.

I make a concerted effort to find paragraphs and short stories that are interesting, so that these clients can practice fluency and increase comprehension. The newspapers published by New Readers Press called *News For You* are practical tools at this time. Edition A is well written on the fourth- to fifth-grade level. Other materials with adult interest are available at lower grade levels. The clients should be reading some of this material every day and should be spending at least one hour a day working on reading skills. This should be designed so that it will be as enjoyable and successful as possible. The various workbooks published for use with aphasic patients are quite helpful at this level and with the lower level reading skills.

Although I will want the client to concentrate on silent reading comprehension, reading aloud in my presence is done frequently. If the reader appears to be trying to read too fast or is overwhelmed by too many words at once, I may make a card with a "word window," allowing only a certain amount of material to be seen at one time. Error types must be defined and the client must be taught to anticipate and to monitor those mistakes. It takes very few errors to completely obscure the meaning of a paragraph!

I believe that this client can also profit from use of the comprehension and speed exercises available from Ann Arbor Publishers in their reading series. These reusable workbooks help the person work on increasing speed of perception and on scanning techniques. It helps accomplish this while avoiding getting bogged down in meaning. I have found the Symbol Discrimination, Symbol Discrimination and Sequencing, and Letter Tracking series particularly effective for meeting these goals. I have also found these workbooks to be beneficial with more severe deficits in teaching left-to-right sequencing and for practice with the alphabet.

In writing, I ask the client to work independently on building vocabulary by doing individual work on spelling words that cause difficulty in reading assignments and other writing assignments. Copying out, spelling aloud, writing from memory, rechecking, and then writing the word in a sentence sequence may help strengthen memory for the correct spelling.

Clients should be formulating sentences using words given by the clinician. They should be encouraged to work on certain grammatical constructions which are particularly troublesome (questions, negatives, etc.) For some, I may wish to pattern the sentences (or a certain form) and gradually decrease the amount of written information given. For example, I may use fill-in-the-blanks for questions, as in "What is your _____?" The pattern may then be continued using the client's wording, and the final task may be to write three questions using "What?"

With more fluent speakers, writing often contains many paragraphic errors, and monitoring of these seems an almost unmanageable task. Monitoring tasks such as having them compare my writing (placed immediately below) to their own may facilitate development of this skill. Finding errors in writing other than their own is also sometimes an effective method.

THE CLIENT WITH A MILD DEFICIT

Persons with a mild deficit in reading and writing demonstrate good reading comprehension on a grade level at, or only slightly below, the premorbid level as long as they are permitted to read very slowly. Short or simple items may be read competently and rapidly, but the longer, more complex, passages must be read slowly if they are to be fully comprehended and stored in memory. In writing, the problem is similar. Writing must usually be very deliberate to be correct. There are frequent spelling errors, and formulation of thought for translation to paper is so slow as to be laborious.

I have found adaptation of some of the techniques used in speed reading courses to be useful for these clients. I have been particularly dependent on a book entitled *How To Read Better and Faster* (Lewis, 1958), although almost any text used in the speed reading courses would probably be similar. The drills in the book called "perception exercises" help the reader focus on a particular point and recognize more and more material in one glance. It eventually enables the person to move along the line faster and to scan with more accuracy. Many of the aphasic clients have the same poor habits that non-brain-injured poor readers display, which slow them down tremendously.

Along with the perception exercises, the client is forced to take material of gradually increasing difficulty and try to read it faster and faster with each trial. I test comprehension with yes/no questions and with specific questions. Clients are repeatedly shown where important points were overlooked and too much time spent on unimportant ideas and "fillers" in the material. They may be asked to go through a paragraph and underline the important points. I gradually fade this activity and let them mentally underscore the important points.

The letter-tracking and thought-tracking activity books from Ann Arbor Publishers are beneficial to these clients, as they push for speed. The workbook series called *Critical Reading* is helpful as it requires the reader to determine whether or not facts have been presented. The reader is constantly appraising the text for fact versus propaganda.

Scanning is encouraged, and I use activities such as looking down a list and finding target items as fast as possible. The phone book provides great material for this activity. The client may be given a certain fact to find and asked to scan text to answer the question. I constantly discourage the client from reading aloud. This slows reading tremendously. If a part of the text is not making sense, then reading it aloud may aid in comprehension. Otherwise, it merely slows the reading process. I watch the client closely for any lip movement that indicates that the words are being said as they are read.

This client must do reading assignments faithfully every day and must spend a significant amount of time each day (average of two to three hours) on reading and writing tasks. Only with this expenditure of effort will success be met. The client may report to me that good work and concentration are very difficult with any auditory distraction in the room. If this is the case, I encourage the client to begin working with a radio playing music. The volume should be increased over time. Radio programs with verbal discourse may then be used. Clients should try to use desensitization to the point that they can read for pleasure in a situation such as a noisy airport waiting area.

The writing assignments must be designed so as to both challenge clients and a level of performance at less than automatic response. The *Workbook for Aphasia* by Brubaker (1978) has numerous activities for writing that are at this level. It also contains good activities for increasing speed of response in higher-level activities that seem almost academically oriented.

The client should be writing letters or some kind of text every day. Reading a newspaper article or short story and then condensing it into one's own words is an excellent activity. This client will many times have difficulty with specificity and may need practice in outlining, to narrow the focus of writing. Practice in note-taking is also beneficial because of the need to select the main points from what one hears or reads and to put it on paper very rapidly.

EVALUATING SUCCESS

The success of a program for the training of reading and writing can be measured by tests that show that the client's performance is improving by a grade level criterion in reading. Standard aphasia tests will also help measure the progress. Measures of reading rate versus comprehension are also good indicators of improvement. The client's own report of enjoyment and success in daily reading and writing is quite an important estimate of progress. If the program has not achieved any measurable progress in a period of one to two months, and the client is reporting no change, I examine methodology closely. There may be a need to redesign the program or to shift goals to a lower level. It is also possible that the client's reading and writing skills have plateaued and that treatment will not make a difference. At this point, I find it best to be honest. Strengths and skills that are present should be emphasized, and compensations for deficits should be discussed. Poor readers may avail themselves of "talking books," available in many cities through the public library, or through services for the visually handicapped. Correspondence can be handled by dictating to a relative or friend if verbal expression is good enough. These are options that are not obvious to everyone. Many clients are quite relieved to know that their struggle can be eased by use of such tactics.

SELECTED REFERENCES

Adult Basic Education and Continuing Education Series. Ann Arbor Publishers, P.O. Box 7249, Naples, Florida 33940.

Brubaker, S. *Workbook for Aphasia.* Detroit: Wayne State University Press, 1978.

LaPointe, L. Aphasia therapy: Some principles and strategies for treatment. In D. Johns (Ed.) *Clinical Management of Neurogenic Communicative Disorders.* Boston: Little, Brown & Co., 1978.

LaPointe, L. Diagnosis and Treatment of Reading Disturbances Associated with Aphasia. Paper presented at the Third Annual Course in Behavioral Neurology and Neuropsychology, Lake Buena Vista, Florida, 1977.

News for You. New Readers Press, P.O. Box 131, Syracuse, N.Y. 13210.

Reading Skills Builders. Readers Digest Services, Educational Division, Pleasantville, N.Y. 10570.

CHAPTER EIGHT

TREATMENT OF ALEXIA WITHOUT AGRAPHIA

Method of Leonard L. LaPointe
and Iris Tanney Kraemer

Alexia without agraphia, or acquired reading impairment with preserved ability to write, is a dramatic though somewhat rare finding in people who have suffered brain damage. As early as 1588, the Italian healer Girolamo Mercuriale wrote that he had discovered "a truly astonishing thing: this man could write but could not read what he had written." However, it remained for the French neurologist Dejerine to elaborate on the nature of this disorder. In two landmark case reports, in 1891 and 1892, Dejerine significantly advanced our knowledge of acquired reading impairment. His punctilious observations of behavior were complemented by autopsy data that provided the first glimmer of understanding regarding the neuroanatomic correlates of reading disruption.

Written language dates back 5,000 years, and the more general condition of alexia, the acquired inability to comprehend written language, has been recognized for centuries. But only in the twentieth century has literacy become sufficiently widespread for acquired alexia to be a significant, recognized problem. In ancient days, very few racks of paperback books existed, and perhaps the only alexia-induced inconvenience in the daily life of prehistoric Java Man was the misinterpretation of directions from cave wall pictographs. To many people in contemporary society, however, impairment of reading ability devastatingly alters quality of life and is more than just a bothersome residual of aphasia.

Purists would argue that the term "aphasia" means total loss of language, while "dysphasia" should be reserved for degrees of impairment short of total loss. Popular and continued usage in the scientific literature has made this distinction somewhat pedantic, however, and these days, "aphasia" is recognized by nearly all as any degree of language loss caused by brain damage. We feel the same way about "alexia" and "dyslexia," and use them interchangably to refer to *degrees* of reading impairment. Acquired alexia, or dyslexia, occurs in the individual whose ability to read was present and became impaired after brain damage; developmental dyslexia refers to an inability to learn to read normally, and is usually discovered during childhood. The principles and approaches used in treatment of developmental dyslexia may or may not be appropriate for acquired dyslexia. Treatment of adults who were once able to read may focus more on facilitation and deblocking strategies than on re-education or acquisition of new skills. Furthermore (and an important point), most reading tests and materials designed for children are inappropriate to adult interests. Puppies, clowns, and balloons should not permeate the subject matter in adult reading material. Most adults would not lament the allocation of Spot and Puff to the humane society.

Another consideration is that the term "reading," in the definition of alexia, refers to the *comprehension* of written material. Loss or impairment of the ability to read aloud without disturbance of the ability to comprehend written language is not alexia.

A rich variety of terms and classification systems have described the varieties of alexia, as can be seen in Table 1. This list is representative, but certainly not exhaustive.

We believe that a brief discussion of the pathogenesis of the condition, along with principles and strategies of evaluation, will aid us in delimiting the nature of alexia without agraphia and subsequently aid us in more effectively presenting the focus of our treatment.

PATHOGENESIS OF ALEXIA WITHOUT AGRAPHIA

A variety of neuropathologies such as tumor, vascular disruption, traumatic head injury, disease, and toxic processes can result in language and reading impairment, but it takes a very specific and clearly defined interhemispheric disconnection to create alexia without agraphia. This syndrome has been repeatedly associated in the literature with cerebral infarction in the distribution of the dominant (usually left) *posterior* cerebral artery. Most commonly, the disconnection necessary to create the syndrome occurs from damage to

TABLE 1 Terminology of Acquired Reading Disturbance

Pure word blindness	Optic alexia
Pure letter blindness	Occipital alexia
Strephosymbolia	Agnostic alexia
Perceptive alexia	Frontal alexia
Semantic alexia	Aphasic alexia
Literal alexia	Central alexia
Tertiary alexia	Pseudoalexia

the left medial occipital lobe of the cortex *and* in the splenium or posterior section of the corpus collosum, that rich bundle of fibers that allows transfer of information between the left and right hemispheres. In essence, the syndrome represents disconnection of the visual-verbal pathways (occipital association cortex from the dominant [left] angular gyrus). The damaged left occipital visual association area prevents appreciation of written or printed material, and the coexisting lesion in the splenium of the corpus collosum prevents transfer of information and blocks participation by the intact visual association areas of the right hemisphere.

ASSOCIATED NEUROLOGIC AND BEHAVIORAL DEFICITS

Since the lesions that create this syndrome are usually vascular and can affect all areas in the distribution of the posterior cerebral artery, we can expect deterioration not only in the visual association area, but in other parts of the neighborhood as well. Many patients will present a right visual field deficit. Paralysis or weakness of the extremities is usually conspicuous by its absence, as is hemisensory loss, except in cases where a portion of the thalamus is involved.

Certain behavioral impairments are frequently associated with the condition. One that occurs most often is color agnosia, or the inability to name colors presented visually. Equally difficult is the task of pointing to colors named by the examiner. Interestingly, people with this disorder have no problem with color names in conversation or by auditory comprehension (e.g., "what color is mustard?"). Verbal memory impairment also accompanies the syndrome and in some patients is severe. Other conditions that have been reported include mild anomia in speech, abnormal written calculation, difficulty in number naming, and occasionally impaired musical notation reading.

READING ERROR TYPES

A number of distinctive patterns or types of errors can be made by people with alexia. "Visual dyslexia" results when errors are caused by confusions of words or letters that are graphically similar. The d/b confusion as in "dug" for "bug" is an example, as well as reversals such as "saw" for "was." "Surface dyslexia," or "grapheme-phoneme dyslexia," is caused by a breakdown in the application of grapheme-phoneme rules. The problem lies in translating a letter to its corresponding sound or phoneme, as in reading "face" for "phase."

"Deep dyslexia," or "syntactic-semantic dyslexia," consists of paraphasias or semantic confusions. Words are read through recognition of their associated meaning, such as "parrot" for "canary" and "sick" for "ill." One patient was described as reading the word "living-room" as "the place we go after dinner to watch T.V." Other more esoteric error patterns may exist, but those just mentioned seem to be the most frequent.

EVALUATION STRATEGIES

Usually the syndrome of alexia without agraphia becomes apparent during the administration of a standard aphasia battery when the marked contrast between reading and writing performance is noted. In order to discern pattern of reading impairment and plan efficient intervention, we make a more detailed assessment of reading.

Several reasons dictate a separate and thorough evaluation of reading. Specific evaluation of reading will allow us to:

1. obtain reading baseline data in order to demonstrate change over time;
2. select appropriate treatment levels and materials; and
3. determine whether or not reading level is functional or adequate for daily living activities.

Standardized Reading Tests

Few standardized reading tests suitable to adult interests are available. Careful evaluation of those that do exist is necessary before they can be used or adapted for adults with brain damage. Many reading tests are not very comprehensive, and a good proportion of them contain juvenile material, which may be inappropriate or demeaning for adults. Tests should be comprehensive and should allow evaluation of both the speed (how much material can be processed in a given period of time) and power (the complexity level at which comprehension breaks down).

The *Reading Comprehension Battery for Aphasia* (RCBA), published by LaPointe and Horner in 1979, allows for a quantitative analysis of reading performance breakdown on the dimensions of accuracy and speed. A number of linguistic, and other factors were considered in selecting the stimulus items for the test, including form class, picturability, frequency, length, reading level, and orthographic and semantic features. The RCBA contains ten subtests that range from matching printed words and pictures to paragraph comprehension. If the RCBA is used to evaluate reading, suggestions on interpreting performance and constructing treatment tasks are contained in the test manual.

INTERPRETATION AND TREATMENT PLANNING

It is sometimes difficult to determine the precise degree of a person's reading loss. In addition to information gathered from the patient's history and family members, reading test performance may be compared with premorbid reading level as estimated by educational and vocational achievement levels.

Performance on the RCBA and the results from the reading sections of aphasia tests, such as the *Boston Diagnostic Aphasia Exam* or the *Minnesota Test for the Differential Diagnosis of Aphasia,* can be used to determine the types of errors made by an individual. These results also can aid in error analysis and the construction of tasks and selection of materials for treatment. Because we are interested in practical, effective, and theoretically sound intervention strategies, we must ask not only how much, and where, but also why performance breaks down.

TREATMENT PRINCIPLES

We use many of the same general approaches for treating other aspects of language impairment in the aphasic person in our treatment of alexia without agraphia. Table 2 lists some of the principles of treatment that guide our work with acquired reading impairment.

Treatment plans are individualized and constructed by evaluating deficit and communicative needs of each patient. Material for tasks is chosen at a level where the patient can usually respond correctly, but with some errors. We find 60 to 80 percent correct response rate is usually a good range within which to construct tasks. The length and complexity of the material is gradually increased as improvement takes place. Objectives are operationalized, baseline behavior is measured, and progress is quantified.

In our clinic, the measurement and quantification of change in communication behavior is an important aspect of treatment. We

TABLE 2 Treatment Principles in Alexia

1. Determine communicative need and importance of reading for each individual.
2. Determine error types or patterns and arrange in treatment priorities.
3. Avoid phonic approach if confounded by paraphasia, auditory impairment, or motor speech deficit.
4. Emphasize comprehension or rate, not oral reading skills.
5. Use material compatible with adult interests.
6. Select functional, daily survival reading tasks for the severely impaired.
7. Construct a reading task continuum; upgrade level with progress.
8. Measure change by probes and retests; chart and plot progress.

use the BASE-10 Response Form as an aid to this objective. Tasks are clearly defined, target levels on each task are determined and specified, stimulus items are selected and entered, and three baselines of performances are measured before instituting treatment. At the beginning of each session, we measure performance on all items prior to the drill or practice on error items, and the resulting score is converted to percentage and entered on a graph that allows visual inspection of sequential progress over ten sessions.

Concentration on reading found in the natural environment and selection of functional tasks relevant to each individual should be a vital element in the selection and construction of reading tasks. Materials we find useful for reading treatment include newspaper and magazine articles, the telephone directory, TV Guide, public building and traffic signs, maps, advertising, menus, recipes, package labels, coupons, meters and gauges, medicine labels, letters and mail, checkbooks, and any other reading requirements we encounter and take so much for granted in our daily wanderings.

SPECIFIC TREATMENT APPROACHES

Comprehension

Treatment for people with alexia without agraphia is not much different from treatment designed for the other types of acquired alexia. For the patient with preserved writing, however, there may be more emphasis on facilitation and deblocking tasks that attempt to capitalize on the relatively intact writing channel.

Since the auditory-verbal connection is intact in alexia without agraphia, patients can immediately recognize a word spelled aloud by the clinician. This preserved recognition of spelled words can sometimes be used to gradually aid recognition of printed words. After demonstrating that spelled words can be recognized, we can design tasks that require the patient to attempt to recognize individual letters and name them aloud. After some proficiency in naming letters has been achieved (this may be tedious and progress may be very slow for the person with letter, or literal, alexia), tasks can be constructed on which the patient attempts to name the letters of short words as he writes them. This deblocking process can be extended until performance on naming individual letters, with subsequent reading of the word, is done rapidly. Gradual fading of the dependence on reading each letter aloud is the objective at this stage of treatment.

The patient with alexia without agraphia also has other modalities that may facilitate deciphering the printed word. Most can recognize individual letters or words when traced on the hand or manually manipulated from embossed blocks. This feature and some of the other preserved functions suggest that what is lost is not the power to associate previously learned concepts with words *per se,* but rather that the access of visual stimuli to the language areas of the brain is compromised, limited, or lost. Deblocking tasks can be constructed that use the facilitating effects of these preserved abilities to recognize embossed, sandpapered, or kinesthetically traced letters and words. As with the tasks that use the intact auditory-verbal loop of letter recognition, the ultimate goal is to fade the dependence on recognition through the modalities of touch, and increase speed and accuracy of recognition and comprehension through the visual mode alone.

With these facilitative or compensatory strategies, progress will be slow and may ultimately end only in the achievement of a labored, compensated style of reading; but surely this is better than no reading at all. The patient who can decipher (no matter how laboriously and compensated) a sign at the zoo that says DO NOT ENTER; HUGE, EMOTIONALLY DISTURBED SNAKES would no doubt welcome his newly acquired reading ability.

Another feature of some patients with this syndrome is the preserved ability to recognize over-learned, very frequently occurring words, such as the name of their city or state, their own name, "USA," "United States," "Coca-Cola," "7-Up," or "Schlitz." Lists of these key words can be assembled and used to attempt to facilitate the recognition of uncomprehended, but similar, words and phrases.

With a technique described as the Visual-Motor Method, the patient is required to write a word from memory. If the written word is incorrect, we repeat the procedure. The patient then attempts to say aloud the word written. We may have to cue, by spelling the word aloud. When the word is reproduced and read accurately, it must be written several more times, covering each previous sample to make sure it is recalled from memory rather than copied. Another word is then introduced, and the procedure is repeated. After a period of time, the words are reviewed.

Manipulation of the physical characteristics of stimuli can be used to facilitate comprehension with some patients. Saliency or the importance of words may be influenced by informational significance, phonologic prominence, or affective-emotional value. The actual size of the stimulus may change performance. For some alexic patients, an increase in the size of the stimulus reduces response time in word reading. Print size, the use of color, and physical prominence are important factors we can systematically alter to influence more accurate reading.

Manipulation of syntactic and semantic features also affects reading. Stimulus sentences that are linguistically less complex result in improved reading speed and comprehension in many patients. Tasks also can be designed around such manipulation of features as the frequency of word usage, the length and number of units in a passage, and amount of exposure time.

Reading Rate Improvement

Multiple Oral Rereading is a technique for increasing reading speed for use in the later stages of a treatment program or for use with mildly involved individuals. This is repeated oral reading of passages selected at the appropriate reading and content level. At each session a new selection, approximately 600 words in length, is read aloud by the patient and timed by a clinician. The assigned selection is then practiced regularly at home between sessions. We find that practice of approximately 30 minutes per day, consisting simply of repeated oral reading of the assigned selection, has been used to increase both speed and fluency.

Not much exists in the literature to guide us in treating any of the syndromes of acquired alexia, let alone specific disorders such as alexia without agraphia. We can only use our clinical acumen and experience, ingenuity, and careful synthesis and application of principles useful in treating other areas of disturbed communication to aid us in managing people with these disorders. Perhaps future empirical research will give us a clearer path. In the meantime, we have at least attempted to blaze a few trees in our outline of some of the principles and strategies found useful in restoring understanding and appreciation of the printed word to people deprived of this enchantment.

SELECTED REFERENCES

Benson, D. and Geschwind, N. The alexias. In P. Vinken and G. Bruyn (Eds.), *Handbook of Clinical Neurology: Disorders of Speech, Perception, and Symbolic Behavior.* New York: American Elsevier, 1969 (pp. 112–140).

Marshall, J. and Newcombe, F. Patterns of paralexia: a psycholinguistic approach. *Journal of Psycholinguistic Research,* 1973 *1:*175–199.

Moyer, S. Rehabilitation of alexia: A case study. *Cortex,* 1979, *15:*139–144.

LaPointe, and Horner, J. *Reading Comprehension Battery for Aphasia.* Tigard, Oregon: C.C. Publications, 1979.

Porazzo, S. Evaluation and treatment of reading deficits in aphasic patients. R. Brookshire, (Ed.), *Clinical Aphasiology Conference Proceedings,* Minneapolis: BRK Pub., 1975.

CHAPTER NINE

TREATMENT OF TRANSCORTICAL MOTOR APHASIA

Method of Michael G. Johnson

DEFINING TREATMENT PARAMETERS

Transcortical motor aphasia, also referred to as anterior isolation syndrome or frontal dynamic aphasia, presents an unusual form of communication disorder. It is primarily characterized by a disturbance of spontaneous speech while speech productions elicited by external stimuli are proportionately better. Speech tends to be free from disturbances in articulation and grammatical errors. An important distinguishing feature is the ability to repeat long, complex sentences, while conversational speech attempts and responses to requests for narrative descriptions are typically limited to one- or two-word responses. Ability to complete sentences, perform series speech, recite familiar passages or rhymes, read aloud, and name items may approach normal. Echolalia may be present, and there may be an inability to inhibit verbal responses under certain conditions. Written productions are often severely distorted early after onset. When legibility returns, written productions can be seen to closely parallel those of speech. It is very important to note that comprehension of spoken or printed material is most often thought to approximate normal. Disturbance of memory, per se, is not associated with transcortical motor aphasia and, therefore, comments such as "I forgot" or "I don't remember" more likely represent an inability to initiate a required response.

Prognosis for transcortical motor aphasia is suggested by existing literature to be very favorable, to the extent that spontaneous conversational speech may return within two to three months. However, I have encountered patients at nine or more months post onset who are unable to respond by virtually any modality without considerable assistance in establishing a response mode. Provided such assistance in the form of treatment, improvements may be dramatic, and a minimum expectation should be fairly reliable responsive speech production abilities.

There are several concomitant behaviors that have been observed with transcortical motor aphasia, most likely due to damage in the vicinity of the superior and mesial premotor area. This area has been

87

shown to be integral in governing the initiation, continuation, and inhibition of (at least) speech. The concomitant behaviors are worthy of mention as they are likely to prove helpful in recognizing the syndrome. Recognition of the syndrome is important, as symptoms closely resemble those seen as a result of diffuse cerebrovascular disease or nonspecific dementia, circumstances wherein prognosis for speech or language disturbances may be considerably less favorable. Furthermore, the following symptoms frequently deserve attention in effective programming of treatment strategies.

Hypokinesis. There will be a noticeable overall hypokinetic state. Lack of spontaneity in speech might easily be interpreted to be the result of an affective disturbance. However, close observation of the patient will reveal an individual who is highly attentive, anxious, often embarrassed, and obviously perplexed by symptomatic behaviors.

Incontinence. There may be incontinence of bowel and/or bladder. This, however, is the direct result of lesion effects on sphincter control rather than inattention or indifference. The incontinence may last for several weeks—again, to the obvious embarrassment of the patient.

Abnormal Vocal Responses. A tendency to cry, unrelated to situational difficulty, may be observed, but the patient is likely to react with puzzlement. When questioned to the effect "Do you really feel like crying?" the response will be denial of feeling sad.

Similarly, the patient may be unable to restrain certain verbal responses. One patient was asked in routine fashion, "How are you today?" to which he immediately responded, "What the h__ do you care!" He immediately shook his head from side-to-side and his face reddened. Such a patient may be unable to refrain from completing a series of numbers or a sentence, even when specifically instructed to remain silent.

Oral Motor Abnormalities. The patient may be unable to perform any oral motor activities, particularly to command. There may be an inability to smile, to produce phonation (even during laughter), or to initiate a swallow, none of which are due to muscular weakness. Conversely, there may be unmitigated vocalizations in the form of "moaning" during normal respirations.

Upper Extremity Abnormalities. There is likely to be proximal weakness (versus more common distal weakness) of the right, upper extremity. Even though weakness at the shoulder may be significant, finger dexterity may approach normal in the right hand. A grasp reflex contralateral to the lesion is common. Movement of either upper extremity may be grossly awkward.

Awareness of limb involvements is important in that limb movements are frequently required in response to evaluation or treatment task instructions. Observations from two cases are presented here for exemplary purposes. Both had confirmed lesions in the distribution of the anterior cerebral artery.

In each case, seating was at a table covered with an array of common objects. There was a tendency for the left, "uninvolved" hand to slowly, but spontaneously reach for an object. When given a verbal command, "Show me what you do with that," there would be uninterpretable movement of the left hand. The left hand then passed the object to the right hand at midpoint in relation to the body. The right hand would grasp the object, volitionally or reflexively, whereupon the two extremities would engage in tugging at the object or aimlessly passing it from one hand to the other, all to the exasperation of the patient. It has been observed that the midpoint in relation to the patient's body serves as an area wherein neither hand is able to decisively grasp and pick up an object. That is, if an object is placed at midpoint, one hand will approach the object, then retreat while the other hand comes near the object, neither of them actually picking up the object. Should one hand pick up the object, competition between hands may again ensue. Each hand tends to restrict its activities to its respective side of the body, never crossing midpoint. Similar performances will be noted in other manipulative tasks, such as when required to place cards (on which printed names of objects appear) on or near objects.

It is important for me to note during such performances that the patient becomes exceedingly bewildered and frustrated. During the course of such peculiar behaviors, full attention of the patient is diverted to the manual activities while another specific task requirement may become lost. I am highly sensitive to such behaviors and their interactions during attempted assessments of comprehension abilities and during the design or implementation of treatment tasks.

ASSUMPTIONS OF TREATMENT

The extent to which transcortical motor aphasia represents a language disorder remains a matter for conjecture. While it is generally agreed that comprehension abilities are well preserved, it is clear that motoric behaviors may be severely restricted. Treatment of the communication disorders associated with transcortical motor aphasia must take into consideration each of the potential symptomatic motor components. It is the distinct impression here that each behavior may require attention in the treatment process; that each observed symptom is integrally related within a symptom complex that results from primary motor processing difficulties. These processing difficulties affect the volitional initiation of motoric responses, maintenance of a required motor act, and/or voluntary inhibition or termination of motor acts. Improvement in speech production may be the primary objective of treatment, but the approach should consider the speech difficulties as one symptom of a broader complex of symptoms that result from overall motor processing difficulties.

In the design of a treatment strategy, I consider the extent to which each observed symptom in the overall complex of motor processing difficulties contributes to decreased speech production. For example, unpredictable crying or aberrant activity of the upper extremities may seriously distract from a primary treatment objective, producing speech. Under such a circumstance, treatment of the crying or limb movements should precede attempts to improve speech production.

Given the assumption that the motor processing problems are functionally interrelated, treatment priorities assigned to nonspeech motor activities may contribute significantly to gaining control of motor speech activities, directly or indirectly. That is, as improvements occur in limb movements, it is conceivable that generalized improvements are occurring in overall motor abilities, including speech production; or, as the patient notices improvements in limb movements, there will be increased confidence and motivation applied to subsequent tasks.

One premise of mine is that concern for an underlying language disorder need not be a primary concern at the outset of treatment. The primary objective is to determine an overall strategy for improving motoric processing, with improvement in verbal communication as the ultimate goal. It is helpful to view the potential severity of symptoms along a continuum that might range from virtually no perceptible response to external stimuli, to slight awkwardness or irregularity in motoric acts, including speech production.

PRETREATMENT CONSIDERATIONS

In the most severe cases, confirmation of underlying linguistic competence may present an unusual challenge. In some cases, only an appeal to emotions will elicit a response. For example, "You are really having a difficult time, aren't you?" may elicit tears; a ridiculous riddle may elicit a semblance of a smile or aphonic laughter; a serious anecdote pertaining to a recent disaster as reported in the news may elicit empathetic furrowing of the eyebrows. Each response provides increased assurance that the individual is attentive, is most likely in fact comprehending, will maintain interest, and will expend effort during continuing treatment activities. Equally or more important, as I give increased clinical assurance that basic linguistic competence is present, and as I verbalize understanding of the patient's circumstances, these responses are gratefully received and gain the patient's confidence in ensuing treatment activities.

Early identification of the transcortical motor aphasia syndrome is my first objective in treatment. It is speculated that the syndrome is frequently misinterpreted as global aphasia due to the patient's inability to respond motorically. Proper and early identification of the syndrome will allow for appropriate education of the patient, the family, and the direct care staff, as well as for disposition and treatment planning in the best interest of the patient.

When involvements are severe and little or no response is consistently observed in verbal or gestural spheres, I direct initial treatment efforts at improving manual/gestural performances. Application of treatment strategies to the upper extremities presents several advantages over oral, pharyngeal, or laryngeal applications. The responses are more visible and readily manipulatable, and improved limb performances very likely contribute to later facilitation of oral-verbal behaviors.

In the absence of significant upper extremity paresis, the more responsive upper extremity should be given preference for executing treatment tasks. The more responsive upper extremity can be identified through performance of a range of limb movements that include gross and fine motor activities. Examples of gross movements are "Pound on the desk," or "Raise your arm all the way up." Examples of fine movements are "Wind a clock," or "Snap your fingers." Each may have to be repeatedly demonstrated to the extent that I must physically manipulate the extremity of the patient in order for it to perform the correct motion on initial trials.

Through the patient's performance, I carefully observe the limb not under performance to determine whether it is typically at rest, or randomly activating in nonpurposeful or distracting activity, or attempting to compete with the performance of the other limb. The degree of effort being expended is also monitored by observing facial expressions or struggle-like tremors of the limb under performance, or by other means. Each observation may assist in defining which limb is more responsive to planned tasks. Treatment activities might necessarily be effected with one upper extremity, then the other, over a number of sessions prior to selecting the upper extremity that will be used consistently through the completion of treatment.

AN APPROACH TO TREATMENT

Phase I: Object-Related Gestures Without Verbalization

1. Introduction. I briefly explain task criteria, emphasizing that no speaking is allowed throughout. Instruction in a few gross, conventional movements is given, such as "Raise your arm way up," "Make a fist," "Salute," or "Wave good-bye." Each is demonstrated, the patient performs them simultaneously with me, then performs each to command with assistance from me as necessary. The purpose, here, is only to convey the general idea of what is expected, not to perfect and differentiate each movement. When this is accomplished, proceed to step two.

2. Simultaneous, imitative use of actual, heterogeneous objects. I place a single object and an identical object before the patient. Example: I state, "Show me how you throw a ball," and both pick up the ball and perform the stated action simultaneously. We both place the ball back on the table. The command-action sequence is repeated until I am assured that the patient is performing the movement with relative ease.

3. Performance of required movement to spoken command. Example: I state, "Show me how you throw a ball." The patient is required to pick up the ball and demonstrate a throwing motion, then return the ball to the table. The steps are repeated until the required movements are performed easily.

4. Patient pantomimes the required movement, actual object, or pictured object present. Example: I state, "Show me how you throw a ball." The patient must perform the required movement without touching the actual object.

5. Patient pantomimes required movement without actual or picture object present. Example: I state, "Show me how you throw a ball." The patient performs the required movement without any additional visual information.

6. Patient pantomimes required movement, action not stated by me. Example: I state, "Show me what you do with this (pointing to actual object or pictured object)." The patient performs the required movement. I use a single object throughout each step at the outset of treatment, thereby reinforcing response requirements for each object. Following completion of all steps with a single object, I proceed through each preceding step with a second object, one that requires a very heterogeneous movement by comparison to the preceding object.

7. Patient pantomimes required movement following a specific command, with two (or more) objects before the patient. Example:

I state, "Show me how you throw a ball." I then state "Show me how you stir coffee with a spoon." I alternate between the two objects until it is assured the patient can simultaneously perform each activity without difficulty. I proceed through each step with additional, heterogeneous objects until at least five have been mastered, then I proceed to the next step.

8. Patient pantomimes required movement in response to command, with no objects or pictured objects present. Example: I state, "Show me what you do with a ball," proceeding through each of the five objects mastered to this point. I revert to previous steps as necessary for any of the items presented in order to accomplish required movements for each of the five objects, alternately.

The difficulty of the foregoing steps may be increased in a variety of ways including:

a. As the number of items mastered increases beyond five, step 7 may be modified by replacing each object with another previously mastered object, thereby rotating objects and movements through the universe of available objects.

b. Gross motor movements tend to be easier than fine motor movements, e.g., throwing a ball versus winding a clock.

c. Step 7 can include objects with homogeneous movements within the array, e.g., key, light bulb, spoon (for stirring), clock, screwdriver; knife, saw, toothbrush, whisk broom, dust cloth.

d. Step 7 or step 8 may be increased in difficulty by requiring the response to occur within a reduced time frame, e.g., within three versus five seconds; then within two seconds, as performance noticeably improves. Initially, it may be necessary to encourage a delay prior to responding to reduce the probability of perseverative responses.

e. Initial treatment criteria may allow gross (but accurate) movements to occur, whereas subsequent sessions require exacting, refined movements. For example, it is common to see large, semicircular movement at the wrist in response to dialing a telephone. The movement should ultimately require reduced wrist movement, increased index finger movement in a semicircular pattern, clockwise, not to exceed the approximate diameter of an actual telephone dial.

Phase II: Conventional Gestures Without Verbalization

The second phase of treatment is pursued when the patient demonstrates accuracy and proficiency in the required movements of at least 20 objects. It is possible that the following phase will be mastered readily, yet it is important to pursue to ensure that the patient does not confine the concept of gestural facilitation to object-related gestures.

I select movements from an array of relatively universal signs (stop, come here, wave good-bye), and utilize those most appropriate to the individual's immediate surroundings or needs.

1. Patient pantomimes the required movement simultaneously with me. Example: I state, "Beckon someone to come closer," while demonstrating the action and assuring that the patient is adequately performing the movements.

2. Patient pantomimes the required movement in response to command. Example: I state, "Show me how to beckon someone to come closer" and wait for the patient's response.

3. Patient pantomimes the required movement in response to a hypothetical situation. Example: I state, "Suppose someone is too far away from you; what do you do?" The patient performs the required movement.

4. Patient pantomimes varied movements in response to hypothetical situations. Additional movements are added to previously performed movements, as in Phase I, Step 7. Additionally, items previously presented in Phase I, Step 8 may be presented here for variety in required responses and for review of previously mastered movements.

Phase III: Verbal Description of Required Movements

This phase is introduced only when the patient demonstrates proficiency in the previous phases of treatment. It is critical in each ensuing step that the required movement occurs prior to verbalization; that there is actual gestural demonstration preceding what is to be conveyed verbally.

1. Patient demonstrates required movement in response to command, then verbalizes what he/she is doing *while* performing the movement. Example: I state, "Show me how you throw a ball." The patient pantomimes throwing a ball. I state, "What are you doing?" The patient again pantomimes throwing a ball, simultaneously stating "I am throwing a ball." (Responses such as "Throwing; I'm throwing; Throwing a ball" should not be accepted as a final product of this step).

2. Patient demonstrates required movement while verbalizing what he/she is doing. Example: I state, "What do you do with this?" while pointing to an object. The clinician must be sure that the

gestural activity is being initiated, and that it is being initiated correctly *prior* to the act of verbalization.

3. Patient demonstrates required movement and verbalizes what he/she is doing in response to hypothetical circumstances. Example: I state, "Someone has poured cream into your coffee. What must you do?" The patient demonstrates a stirring motion while stating "I (must) stir my coffee."

ADDITIONAL CONSIDERATIONS

Each step in the program has precisely defined criteria for: (1) the form of instructions to the patient; (2) adequacy of specificity of the required response (the response must basically be specific enough to differentiate it from other responses); (3) when and how a response perceived to be inadequate is to be terminated in favor of additional instructions or return to a previous step (I interrupt an inaccurate response immediately upon identifying it as incorrect or potentially incorrect); and (4) how each response is to be recorded. At a minimum, the recording system differentiates responses that are correct and prompt, delayed, self-corrected, partially adequate, or the result of additional instructions. Erroneous responses are only accepted when obtaining base line data.

Successful completion of the foregoing phases of treatment is intended to prepare the patient to proceed to more normal verbal behaviors using refined self-cueing methods, such as "imagining" the intended activity to be verbalized before verbalizing. I may try to improve overall rate or prosody of speech, or to reduce perseverative tendencies. Given reliable motor response abilities at this point, it may become evident that more traditional language retraining is of benefit. Primary motor processing disturbances should have been greatly reduced, however, thereby allowing observations of actual, underlying communicative abilities of the patient. Modifications of this program are undoubtedly possible and encouraged. For example, the inclusion of bimanual activities may be of benefit in later phases of programming and are evaluated. The foregoing program is intended to assist in unlocking patients from truly perplexing phenomena. Improvements are typically forthcoming.

SUGGESTED READINGS

Albert, M., Goodglass, H., Helm, N., Rubens, A., and Alexander, M: Dysphasia without repetition disturbance. In *Clinical Aspects of Dysphasia*, New York, Springer-Verlag Wien, 1981.

Rubens, A: Aphasia with infarction in the territory of the anterior cerebral artery. *Cortex*, 1975, *XI*:239–250.

Rubens, A: Transcortical motor aphasia. In H. Whitaker and H. Whitaker (Eds.), *Studies in Neurolinguistics* (Vol. I). New York: Academic Press, Inc., 1976.

CHAPTER TEN

TREATMENT OF SUBCORTICAL APHASIAS

Method of Nancy Helm-Estabrooks

Within the past ten years, several subcortical aphasia syndromes have been described. Among these are thalamic aphasia and the capsular-putamenal aphasias (anterior, posterior, and global).

The introduction of the computed tomographical (CT) brain scan permitted aphasiologists to identify these new aphasias by correlating their predominately subcortical lesion sites with patterns of speech and language behaviors. Prior to CT scanning, these aphasia syndromes were unclassified, because they did not conform to speech/language patterns observed in cortical aphasias, such as Broca's, Wernicke's, and anomic aphasia. Similarly, they did not respond to the treatment approaches developed for patients with cortical lesions. Thus, it became necessary to develop new treatment techniques addressing the specific deficits characteristic of subcortical aphasia syndromes. The development and investigation of treatment approaches is a slow process. The techniques I describe have been used successfully with a handful of patients with subcortical aphasia. They are not pre-scriptions for all subcortical aphasias. They are, however, techniques that I have found to be successful with patients like the two to be described here.

PATIENT DESCRIPTION

Patients A and B had aphasia profiles that appeared essentially "global" at three months post-onset of stroke. Performance was severely impaired on most subtests of the Boston Diagnostic Aphasia Examination. Praxis testing showed severe buccofacial and gestural/limb apraxia. Both patients had a right hemiparesis, with the arm more involved than the leg. CT scanning showed that unlike many global patients with large frontal parietal temporal lesions, A and B had relatively small subcortical lesions that centered in the putamen and internal capsule. Also, unlike many global patients, A and B spontaneously produced a few hypophonic *real* word stereotypies like "this and this," "this thing," "this day." These stereotypies were not communicatively effective. A nonverbal behavior rating scale showed that A and B used no effective gesturing beyond the level of simple pointing.

97

APPROACH I: VISUAL ACTION THERAPY

Both patients were first treated with two forms of Visual Action Therapy (VAT), i.e., "limb" VAT and "face" VAT.

The goal of Visual Action Therapy is to train patients to represent, through gestural symbols, a set of pictured objects that are hidden from view. In "limb" VAT, all eight objects can be represented by hand gestures that move away from the body, while in "face" VAT, all eight objects are represented by movements that involve the face. In a sense, "limb" VAT may be regarded as a treatment for gestural/ limb apraxia, while "face" VAT may treat facial apraxia. In addition, VAT may improve such skills as attention, visual scanning, and visual discrimination.

Visual Action Therapy ("limb" and "face") is a nonverbal, three-level, hierarchically structured program that utilizes (1) eight *unimanual* objects, which can be represented with distinct gestures, (2) large, shaded line drawings of each object on 5" × 8" index cards, (3) small, shaded line drawings of each object on 1½" × 3" cards, and (4) eight 3" × 5" action pictures depicting each object being manipulated by stick figures.

The objects for "limb" VAT are: hammer, saw, screwdriver, paintbrush, section of phone containing dial, doorknob (mounted in wood), salt shaker, and egg whisk. Contextual prompts are used in conjunction with some objects, for example, a piece of wood containing a large nail is used with the hammer, and a bowl with the egg whisk.

Following completion of "limb" VAT, patients receive a course of "face" VAT. The objects for "face" VAT are: cup, whistle, drinking straw, flower, razor, telescope, lollipop, Chapstick.

The following procedure is used both for "limb" VAT and "face" VAT.

General Instructions

Visual Action Therapy is a *nonverbal* method for severely aphasic patients. All directions, reinforcements, and treatment steps are non-verbal. The program follows a hierarchy of difficulty, so that close to 100 percent success is required for each step before moving to the next. The patient's performance with each object at each scorable step is scored 1.0 for fully correct, .5 for self-correct, and 0 for any other behavior. Steps labeled *Training* are unscorable. It is advisable to review the previous, or easier, step at the beginning of new sessions, which last approximately one-half hour.

Although eight objects are generally used, this number may be reduced to as few as four for the most impaired patients.

Step One: Trace Training

The goal of this step is to help the patient understand that *line drawings* of objects can represent, or "stand for," objects. *First,* I trace the patient's hand onto a large piece of unlined paper and color in the outline. *Second,* I help the patient trace my hand on a second piece of paper. *Third,* I help the patient trace two of the objects, e.g., screwdriver and hammer, on pieces of paper. *Fourth,* the line drawings are arranged in front of the patient. *Fifth,* the patient is handed the hammer to place on the correct drawing, then the screwdriver. I then put my hand on the correct line drawing, and finally encourage the patient to place his hand on the remaining drawing.

If the patient is unable to perform this task, I try additional tracing training. If the patient continues to show confusion, this treatment procedure is probably inappropriate, and should be discontinued for the present.

Step Two: Large Picture Matching

Object-to-Picture Matching. All eight large object cards are arranged in a random order line in front of the patient. Each object is randomly handed (one at a time) to the patient, to be placed on the matching picture.

Picture-to-Object Matching. All eight objects are arranged in a random order line in front of the patient, and the aforementioned procedure is repeated with the large object cards.

Picture-to-Object Pointing. All eight objects are randomly arranged in front of the patient. The large object cards are held up, one at a time, for the patient to see. With nonverbal cues, he is instructed to *point* with the index finger to the objects that match the cards. This may require direct manipulation of the patient's hand in order to establish the pointing set.

Object-to-Picture Pointing. All eight large object picture cards are randomly arranged before the patient. The objects are held up one by one and the patient is encouraged to *point* to the matching picture.

Step Three: Small Picture Matching

The same four steps described in Step Two are followed, using the small object picture cards and the eight objects.

Step Four: Object Use Training

Each object is presented one at a time with contextual prompt where indicated. I demonstrate the object's use, e.g., pound the nail with the hammer. The object is then placed in front of the patient, who is encouraged to pick it up and demonstrate the use of the object. If the patient has persistent difficulty manipulating a particular object, a substitute object may be chosen.

Step Five: Action Picture "Command" Training

Each object is presented alone with the matching action picture propped up for the patient to see (usually within the left visual field). I point to the action card, then pick up the object and demonstrate its use (with contextual prompts where indicated). The object is then placed in front of the patient, I point to the action card, and the patient is encouraged to properly manipulate the object.

Step Six: Following Action Picture "Commands"

All eight objects with contextual cues are arranged in front of the patient. One at a time, I hold up any action card and encourage the patient to find the appropriate object and demonstrate its use.

Step Seven: Pantomimed Gesture Demonstration

One by one, each object (without contextual prompts) is placed to the left front of the patient. I then produce the pantomimed gesture that is most commonly associated with the object and can be used to "represent" it.

Step Eight: Pantomimed Gesture Recognition

All eight objects (without contextual prompts) are placed before the patient. I produce a representational gesture for each, and the patient is encouraged to point to the object associated with the gesture.

Step Nine: Pantomimed Gesture Training

All eight objects are placed one by one to the patient's left, and he is encouraged to produce a representational gesture for each. If he fails or has difficulty, I provide assistance until the patient can initiate the gesture. This may involve placing an object in the patient's hand for direct manipulation and then slowly removing it while the appropriate movement is maintained.

Step Ten: Pantomimed Gesture Production

The eight objects are held up to the patient one by one and he is encouraged to produce a representational gesture for each.

Step Eleven: Representational Gesture for Absent Object Training

Two objects at a time are placed in front of the patient, and I produce the appropriate representational gestures for each. The two objects are hidden under a cloth and then one is brought back into view. I produce questioning gestures as if to ask, "What object is still under the cloth?" I then produce the representational gesture associated with the hidden object.

Step Twelve: Representational Gesture for Absent Object Production

Step Eleven is repeated with the patient providing the appropriate representational gesture for hidden objects. Once again, the procedure is for two objects at a time to be presented and hidden, but for only one to remain hidden and represented with a gesture. The process is repeated for each combination of pairs, so that each object remains hidden during this step.

Level II

Steps 7 to 12 of Level I are repeated, with the action cards substituted for the objects.

Level III

Steps 7 to 12 of Level I are repeated, with the small object picture cards substituted for the objects.

Upon completion of "limb" and "face" VAT, Boston Diagnostic Aphasia Examination (BDAE) test scores earned by patients placed them well above the level of global aphasia in the areas of auditory and reading comprehension. Speech output, however, remained limited to a few well-articulated real word stereotypies. Both patients were unable to read aloud any of the words on a BDAE oral reading subtest, though they were able to match words to pictures on another subtest. When presented with printed versions of their own stereotypies, however, both A and B were able to read these words aloud correctly. Therefore, both patients were entered into a second course of treatment, called Voluntary Control of Involuntary Utterances (VCIU) to improve speech output.

APPROACH II: VOLUNTARY CONTROL OF INVOLUNTARY UTTERANCES

Voluntary Control of Involuntary Utterances (VCIU) was developed for patients who produced a few real words either as stereotypies or, occasionally, at random. For example, patient A usually produced the stereotypic phrase "this and this" in conversation, but occasionally uttered "yes" and "no." When asked to repeat *hammock,* he said "kiss." For *W,* he said "two." When asked to name *chair,* he said "die." Oral reading of *fifteen* yielded "three-five."

VCIU begins with a written presentation of any real word the patient has been heard to utter. The appropriateness or correctness of the word is disregarded. If the patient has been heard to utter "kiss" then *kiss* is printed on a 3″ × 5″ note paper for oral reading. Patient A could orally read all of the foregoing words correctly. Because two of the words he had uttered spontaneously have emotional connotation, i.e., *kiss* and *die,* he was presented with similar words, e.g., *love, sick, hate.* If he read these words correctly and immediately, they were retained. If he uttered another real word for the stimulus word, the original stimulus was discarded and the spontaneously uttered real word was substituted. For example, when the stimulus "hi" was read as "hello," *hi* was discarded and *hello* was presented and read correctly. If instead of *hello,* he had said "bye," then that word would have been substituted and *hello* disregarded.

In VCIU, the patient determines the practice lexicon. I initiate the process by offering words that the patient has been heard to say or words that I think the patient might be able to read aloud. Emotion-laden words have proved to be particularly successful.

In our clinic, we keep a master list of words that many of our subcortically aphasic patients have been able to read aloud. This list provides "starters" for similar patients. Some of these high success words are:

ball	no
book	okay
bye	see
coke	shoe
key	show
four	tie
good	time
have	two
I don't know	one
juice	what
love	watch
lunch	wow

If a patient can correctly read a word aloud without struggle, this word is printed in black felt tip pen on a 3″ × 5″ card. This card, along with the others, is given to the patient for self-review outside the clinic. I retain a master list for each patient and add to it during each session.

The next step in VCIU is to present the patient with opportunities to produce the target words correctly in a confrontation and/or responsive-naming mode. If the target word is picturable (e.g., car) or environmental (e.g., door), then we simply ask, "What is this?" If the target word is nonpicturable, then a responsive naming format is used, e.g., for *love* we might ask, "What is the opposite of hate?"

The final step in VCIU is to set up conversational situations which may elicit the target words. For example, by asking a patient if he has ever had a flat tire, and engaging him in conversation about the experience, we provide the conversational opportunity for him to use the words *car, tire, up,* etc., and perhaps a few emotion-laden words.

With both patients A and B, and with similar patients, we have seen a rapid extension of the available verbal repertoire with VCIU. A and B added new words to their lists every session. More importantly, both began to increase their spontaneous speech output to include appropriate and therefore communicative utterances. With a course of VCIU, both patients accumulated hundreds of practice cards and showed improved functional speech skills. Readministration of the BDAE showed improved verbal subtest scores.

SELECTED REFERENCES

Alexander, M. and LoVerme, S. Aphasia after left hemisphere intracerebral hemorrhage. *Neurology,* 1980, *30*:1193–1202.

Helm-Estabrooks, N., Fitzpatrick, P., and Barresi, B. Visual action therapy for global aphasia. *Journal of Speech and Hearing Disorders,* 1982, *47*:385–389.

Helm, N. and Baressi, B. Voluntary control of involuntary utterances: A treatment approach to severe aphasia. In R. Brookshire (Ed.), *Clinical Aphasiology Conference Proceedings.* Minneapolis: BRK Publishers, 1980.

Landis, T., Graves, R., and Goodglass, H. Emotional value facilitates lexical output in aphasia. *Cortex,* 1982, *18*:105–112.

Naeser, M., Alexander, M., Helm, N., Levine, H., Laughlin, S., and Geschwind, N. Aphasia with predominantly subcortical lesion sites: Description of three capsular/putaminal syndromes. *Archives of Neurology,* 1982, *39*:1.

CHAPTER ELEVEN

TREATMENT OF COMMUNICATION DEFICITS RESULTING FROM TRAUMATIC HEAD INJURY

**Method of Brenda L. Adamovich and
Jennifer A. Henderson**

The incidence of head injuries is increasing owing primarily to high-velocity transportation in a fast-paced society. At the same time, mortality rates have declined due to medical and technological advancements. Effects on abilities to communicate are wide ranging, and so are appropriate treatments. If speech, fluency, voice, and/or swallowing deficits occur, we utilize traditional methods of treatment, but not until attention and recall abilities allow for active participation in therapy. Nonvocal communication devices should be considered for head trauma patients who are unable to communicate verbally, provided patients possess the cognitive and physical abilities necessary to utilize these devices. Owing to the frequent occurrence of oral and facial injuries following accidents that cause head trauma, a prosthodontist is often needed, along with rehabilitation programs in conjunction with physical, psychosocial, and behavioral restoration. Patients with aphasia secondary to cortical and subcortical lesions are treated by means of specific techniques outlined in other chapters in this text. Specific language problems can be confused with general cognitive deficits. The level of cognitive functioning must be considered when evaluating and treating specific language disorders. Patients must have selective attention and the ability to remember learned strategies before language therapy is initiated.

The most incapacitating and long-lasting sequelae of accidents in which close head injuries have occurred are cognitive or information-processing difficulties. Patients with confused language (the most common cause of communication difficulty following head trauma) and general intellectual impairments resulting in an overall decline in cognitive processes, including high level linguistic skills, are treated by means of techniques described in this chapter.

105

INFORMATION PROCESSING

Our treatment program focuses on changing and modifying the patient's behavior, followed by the generalization of this behavior to the patient's home and community. To achieve these goals, the patient must be able to learn, retain, and generalize information. Learning a new fact requires the establishment and maintenance of new relationships or links between concepts that are already known. Patients with traumatic head injuries have difficulty integrating, assimilating, and/or accommodating new information. When treating information-processing deficits, we utilize the following four-stage treatment hierarchy: alerting and stimulating, orienting, operative retraining, and self-reliant functioning in the home and community.

ALERTING AND STIMULATING (ATTENTION AND PERCEPTION)

Basic attentional skills are necessary for patients to actively participate in therapy sessions. Improvement of attention is a secondary focus of every task.

We use initial attention and perception tasks to activate a response to any stimulus (tactile, auditory, visual, verbal, gustatory, olfactory, and vestibular) and to gradually increase the frequency, type, and duration of response. Arousal or alerting tends to be dependent upon the strength of the stimulus. Sensory deprivation must be avoided and abnormal reflexes must be decreased.

Specific auditory and verbal stimulation activities include:

1. Auditory stimulation and tracking tasks that progress from the use of gross, nonspeech sounds (bell, buzzers, musical instruments, etc.) to more finely discriminated speech sounds. (We begin with familiar voices, both live and taped, of family members, and progress to unfamiliar voices, including those on the radio and television.)

2. Auditory recognition and perception in which the patient is asked to identify environmental sounds, phonemes, words, and sentences by verbally responding, or by pointing to corresponding pictures or words.

3. Verbal stimulation in which gross, reflexive sounds are elicited first. We gradually work toward vocalizations appropriate to specific situations.

ORIENTATION

We review orientation information with the patient every morning and prior to each therapy session. Specific information reviewed includes: patient's name, name of the facility, day of the week, month, date, year, specific time, the names of each team member, and the time of each therapy appointment. Visual cues are placed in each patient's room to be utilized during the orientation tasks, including: a calendar, clock, bulletin board containing pictures of each team clinician, and a card on which the name of the hospital is printed. A daily appointment schedule is fastened to each patient's wheelchair indicating the time of each appointment.

We also conduct a reality-orientation group. Group activities include: a review of orientation information presented in individual sessions, familiarization with the physical plant of the hospital, and a review of each group member's biographical information.

OPERATIVE RETRAINING

Discrimination

Daily activities require selective attention in which multiple aspects of a stimulus situation must be discriminated at any moment in time. Relevant, irrelevant, and extraneous stimuli must be identified. It is important to note that the salient or pertinent aspects are not necessarily related to the strength or intensity of the stimulus, as in the arousal or alerting activities. During the selective-attention process, the patient must rely on contextual cues. The threshold for highly pertinent information must be continually adjusted.

Our treatment focuses on gradually increasing the number and degree of similarity of stimuli that compete with the most pertinent stimuli. During routine communicative situations, attention is maintained for a period of time during which attention is switched from one message to another and from one stimulus to the next in the same message. Head trauma patients tend to be stimulus-bound. They respond to a salient property of the stimulus and fail to remain oriented to the task.

Specific therapy activities include visual and auditory tasks in which:

1. The patient is to discriminate color, shape, or size by visually matching geometric forms or by pointing to the forms following an

auditory command. Initially, we present only two response items, which differ by only one feature, i.e., same shape, same size, different colors. Gradually, the number of items and the features per response set are increased.

2.   The patient is to visually match objects to objects, followed by pictures to objects, pictures to pictures, letters to letters, words to words, and words to objects. We gradually increase the complexity of the response set by increasing the number of items and the degree of color, shape, size, and function similarities of the response items (e.g., match a pen to a pen in an array of objects including pencil, magic marker, chalk, and pen).

3.   The patient is required to point to objects, pictures, letters, and words by name. We begin with a field of two items and gradually increase the number, as well as the phonemic and semantic similarity, of the response items.

4.   The patient is required to visually match a picture to a sentence. We begin with a field of two items and gradually increase the number of response items.

5.   The patient must auditorily discriminate between words or sentences. When given two visually and/or auditorily similar words (e.g., *cat* and *cot*) or sentences (e.g., *she picked up the dog* or *she picked at the dog*), the patient is to correctly identify the word or sentence given verbally by the clinician.

6.   The patient is required to respond to questions regarding biographical information. Initially, we require yes/no responses (gestures or words) followed by the provision of the actual information by the patient.

7.   The patient is to follow simple commands, e.g., "open your eyes, lower your legs, close your mouth."

Organization

The process of organization plays an important role in the acquisition of new information, in recall, and in other high level processes such as problem solving and logical thinking. The organization of information utilizes learned strategies in which discrete actions or components of stimuli must be organized and sequenced according to the priority of each component.

Specific therapy tasks utilized to improve organization skills include:

1.   Categorization tasks in which:

a. The patient is to visually sort, or give to the clinician upon request, a group of geometric forms by sizes, shapes, and colors. We begin with four items that differ by only one feature, i.e., same size, same color, different shapes, and gradually increase the number of items and stimulus features in each response set.

b. The patient must match items (pictures, letters, words, etc.) that are in the same class but not identical, e.g., match A to a, or match different species of birds.

c. The patient is to sort objects when the categorical set is changed and the same objects are used, e.g., a group of geometric forms are first sorted according to color, followed by shape, then size.

d. We discuss attributes of various geometric shapes, i.e., number of sides, angles, horizontal lines, etc. The patient is given additional shapes, which must be assigned to specific groups based on similarities and differences to other group members.

e. We arbitrarily assign nonsense names to several groups of geometric shapes. The similar and different attributes of each group must be analyzed by the patient in order to assign names to new stimuli presented by the clinician.

f. The patient is required to sort objects into general categories, such as foods, eating utensils, writing implements. etc. Items should then be subdivided into more specific categories, such as fruits, vegetables, meats.

g. The patient is to verbally provide descriptive (physical attributes) and functional (use) similarities and differences between two objects, such as a table and a chair or an orange and a canteloupe.

2. Closure activities in which:

a. Nonlinguistic tasks are presented which require the identification of geometric forms with sections missing, for example:

$\cup$ or $\boxminus$

Next, we present pictures of objects with parts missing, and scenes with objects missing.

b. Visual linguistic tasks are presented which require the identification of words with portions of letters missing, e.g., si\; words with letters missing (last letter should be omitted first, followed by initial letter, then medial letters), e.g., lak_, _ake, l_ke, b_tt_m; sentences with words missing, e.g., John _____ to the store; steps to the completion of a task with one or more steps missing; and paragraphs with sentences missing.

c. Auditory linguistic tasks are presented, such as sound

blending in which phonemes are individually presented, and the patient must identify the word.

3. Sequencing tasks in which:

a. Nonlinguistic tasks are presented requiring the patient to sequence a color from light to dark shades, or objects from small to large.

b. Linguistic tasks are presented requiring the patient to:

(1) connect dots in a numerical or alphabetical order.

(2) reorder (forward and backward) strings of numbers, letters, days of the week, and months of the year.

(3) visually or auditorily sequence words in which letters or syllables are out of order, sentences in which words are scrambled, and paragraphs in which sentences are scrambled.

(4) sequence steps of activities of daily living including washing, eating, shopping.

4. Fragmented stimuli in which:

a. The patient is to correctly assemble stimulus items such as pictures of common objects which are cut into pieces.

b. The patient is to correctly assemble puzzles. We begin with simple puzzles and progress to more complex puzzles.

5. Figure ground tasks in which questions must be answered regarding information presented aurally under various conditions of background noise, e.g., cafeteria conversation, traffic sounds.

6. Daily routines should be organized, such as treatment schedules, placement of articles in the room, and functional tasks, e.g., washing, dressing, cooking, money management, shopping, etc. Initially, we provide order in the patient's environment. The patient should gradually accept the responsibility for establishing this order. A treatment schedule should be prepared by the patient. Articles in the room should be categorized according to function, and steps of each functional task should be identified and sequenced.

Memory

Memory deficits can be long-lasting; therefore, our therapy focuses on providing the patient with strategies to compensate for these deficits. Before we introduce the memory strategies outlined in this section, the patient must achieve competency levels in previous stages of the treatment continuum, including perception, discrimination, and organization of information.

The auditory and visual retention hierarchy is based on the length and amount of information that must be processed, organized, and recalled. Tasks should progress from single items (geometric forms, letters, numbers, and words) to phrases and short sentences, followed by stories and situations. Within each task, item complexity can be increased by considering the following: abstract items are more difficult to recall than concrete items; similar items are more difficult to recall than dissimilar items; items within the task can interfere with the recall of other items within the task, so that similar items preceding the item to be recalled (proactive inhibition), or similar items following the item to be recalled (retroactive inhibition), interfere with the recall; and, unfamiliar and nonmeaningful information is more difficult to recall than familiar information.

We teach memory strategies that facilitate immediate, short-term, and long-term storage and recall of information. Specific strategies include the following:

1. Verbal description in which an adequate explanation of items, concepts, etc. to be recalled is provided by the patient or clinician. In therapy, visual, auditory, and semantic descriptions are encouraged.

2. Visual imagery in which objects, scenes of a story or situation, and maps of layouts in space are mentally pictured.

3. Chunking activities, in which information is organized into segments that coincide with the patient's memory span, e.g., if the patient can recall only two items, information should be divided into two-item segments. When possible, meaningful units are considered when chunking information. When memory is organized into chunks, retrieval of one unit or chunk of information will provide access to more than a single item or relationship. To accomplish chunking, we present stimuli visually with the different segments written in different colors or sizes. The segments can also be physically separated during visual or auditory presentation of the information.

4. Categorization of information to improve recall of that information, e.g., when required to remember 15 items to be purchased at a grocery store, the patient should group the items into categories such as dairy products, frozen foods, meats, etc.

5. Rehearsal in which information to be recalled is drilled, utilizing verbal and visual strategies. Verbal repetition is used in which the information is repeated aloud, subvocally, or silently. Visually, the patient can continually review the details of visual images or written stimuli. Requiring the patient to maintain a daily log of events provides for rehearsal of activities occurring daily and weekly.

6. Associations in which relationships between items or events to be stored or recalled are recognized and accentuated. Associations

can be based on semantic relationships (e.g., cane/crutches and day/night), acoustic relationships (dew/shoe), or visual relationships (desk/dresser).

7. Temporal or spacial ordering in which events in episodic and semantic memory are recalled by remembering certain landmark events associated with the event to be recalled, or which occurred at a similar point in time. Actions or events can often be recalled if the goals or results of the action are recalled. Initially, we emphasize key events during encoding. Using selective reminding during recall, we question and cue patients regarding key events. Gradually the number of cues are reduced.

8. Primacy and recency effects in which the first or last item, respectively, is recalled more often than central items in a string of items. To increase the effects of primacy and recency, the first and last items in a string are accented visually using different colors and sizes, or auditorily, using different loudnesses and pitches.

9. Mnemonic devices in which specific memory tricks are utilized to increase associative learning through paired association. During encoding, new words or bits of information are chained or paired to a pre-established set of key words and phrases or to a familiar sequence of known locations.

High-Level Thought Processes

When teaching cognitive skills, we provide a demonstration and a description rather than a description alone. This technique is particularly important if language skills are impaired. High-level cognitive tasks require the patient to be an active processor of information. Problem-solving or reasoning occurs in several stages: a person must first attempt to understand or analyze the problem; a solution, a strategy, and several alternatives are then formulated based on past experiences stored in long-term memory; next, the solution is generated or executed; and finally, the solution is evaluated. During problem-solving tasks, head trauma patients tend to have a narrow perspective, which results in a concrete and incomplete analysis of problems. They do not take time to think through problems. Patients also have difficulty deciding how to approach the problem. The need for additional information is not recognized, and solutions, therefore, are based on incomplete or partial information.

Our treatment focuses on a variety of problem-solving strategies. When teaching problem-solving techniques, we begin by leading the patient through each step in the process using visual and verbal cues. Next, cues are only provided to keep the patient on target. Finally, the patient is to solve the problem independently. When planning therapy, a hierarchical thought process is considered. Convergent or analytical thinking skills are presented first. Deductive reasoning tasks are introduced second, followed by inductive reasoning and divergent thinking.

Convergent Thinking

During convergent thinking tasks, the patient analyzes information in order to identify the central or main point. This process requires recognition of relevant and irrelevant information. In communicative situations, convergent thinking skills allow an individual to understand and formulate the general theme of a conversation, situation, or written article.

Specific therapy tasks include:

1. The identification of relevant information in visually and/or auditorily presented sentences, paragraphs, and conversations with respect to who did what, when, and where. *The Folkes Sentence Builder* series is helpful for this task.

2. The reduction of information to the most salient items by abstracting the main idea of visually and/or auditorily presented sentences, paragraphs, and conversations. Key facts and situations should be identified by considering the intent of the sender and the interpretation of the receiver.

Deductive Reasoning

Deductive reasoning is a process in which conclusions are drawn from given data or situations based on premises or general principles. This requires an analysis that progresses from the whole situation to specific parts or features. Deductive reasoning is necessary in linguistic and nonlinguistic problem-solving tasks, which require an individual to form conclusions supported by the information given. Specific therapy tasks include:

1. Forward or backward chaining, in which the patient is to deal with the relevant information and devise solutions in a progressive (forward) or regressive (backward) step-by-step process until the final solution is reached. Problems are presented in *Mind Benders: Deductive Thinking Skills,* which requires a forward process of variable elimination. Situational pictures can be given which require a backward

process of variable elimination, e.g., a picture of an accident involving two cars.

2. Missing-premise tasks, in which two facts are necessary to reach a conclusion. If given one fact, the patient is to choose the second fact that leads to the conclusion. (Given: "All children must go to school, and Bob and Jane are children." The patient is to deduce that Bob and Jane must go to school.) The *Ross Test of Higher Cognitive Processes* is especially useful for these tasks.

Inductive Reasoning

Inductive reasoning is a process in which solutions are formulated by considering particular details which lead to, but do not necessarily support, a general conclusion. This requires an analysis of parts or details to formulate an overall, or whole, concept. In communicative situations, a person must analyze given details and gather additional information in order to assess a situation, e.g., in determining whether a call should be placed to the rescue squad, a person must gather information to determine the seriousness of tne situation. Specific therapy tasks include:

1. The formulation of antonyms and synonyms. Crossword puzzles are useful in this task.

2. Analogous thinking in which the patient is given two or more items or pairs of items which must be analyzed with regard to similar or different features in order to provide a word or pair of words related in the same way, e.g., the patient is to respond "cat," if given the statement, "Bark is to dog as meow is to ____."

3. Cause and effect tasks, in which either the cause or the effect of a situation is presented. The patient must indicate the appropriate solution, e.g., if given: "Boiling water is spilled on a woman's hand," the patient is to indicate that the woman's hand is burned; or if given "A woman's hand is burned," the patient is to indicate that the woman's hand came in contact with a source of heat such as boiling water, fire, etc.

4. Open-ended problem solving, including story-completion tasks in which the patient is required to complete an unfinished story.

5. Decision-making tasks, in which a situation is given and the patient is required to make a choice between possible solutions, e.g., if given the problem "John needs money," the patient is to indicate that John should go to work rather than rob a bank (or other possible, but socially unacceptable, solutions).

Divergent Thinking

Divergent thinking results in the generation of unique abstract concepts or hypotheses which deviate from standard concepts or ideas. The hypotheses or concepts must then be tested. Without divergent thinking skills, linguistic and situational paradoxes, abstractions, and subtleties are overlooked, and experiences are often viewed incorrectly due to literal or concrete interpretations.

Specific therapy tasks include:

1.   Multi-meaning stimuli (homographs), in which the patient is required to construct sentences depicting several meanings for each sentence or phrase. Given "shoulder," responses could be: "A shoulder is part of your body," "He drove on the shoulder of the road," or "You don't have to shoulder the burden."

2.   Multi-function stimuli (simile and metaphor formulation and interpretation) requiring the analysis of a figure of speech in which one object or event is described in terms usually denoting another object or event, e.g., "the ship *plowed* the sea." A likeness or analogy between the objects or events is implied, although abstract thinking is required to discern the similarities.

3.   Absurdities in which the patient is to describe what is absurd about statements and stories, such as, "The temperature rose to 25°, so he chipped through the ice and went for a swim."

4.   Idiom interpretation requiring the patient to provide explanations of phrases in which the meaning generally cannot be derived from the literal interpretation of its parts, e.g., *empty-headed, chicken-hearted, clear as mud, on pins and needles.*

5.   Proverb interpretations requiring the patient to analyze a statement in which true, nonstandard abstract meanings and relationships of items are given. The statements can be satirical and/or paradoxical as well as contraindicatory or nonsensical. These truths are of a general rather than specific sense.

6.   The interpretation of poetry, fables, puns, jokes, and riddles which require the patient to consider abstract relations, double meanings, paradoxes, and nonstandard meanings.

Multi-process Reasoning

Multi-process reasoning requires the use of several thought processes previously described. Specific therapy tasks include:

1.   Determining whether or not sufficient, extra, or unnecessary

information has been provided in a given problem. If the information is inadequate to solve the problem, the patient must utilize a questioning strategy to gather necessary information regarding the central features of the problem.

2.   Responding to questions based on an analysis of syllogisms or arguments consisting of a major and a minor premise and a conclusion, e.g., assumptions: (a) if John catches a 5-pound fish, he will win a trophy. (b) If John wins two more trophies this month, he will have won a total of six trophies. (c) John does not catch a 5-pound fish. Questions: (a) Did John win a trophy? (b) Could John win six trophies during this month? Using deductive reasoning, a conclusion is derived by the patient based on the two or more assumptions. In the second, more complex, part of this task, the validity of the conclusion must be determined by means of inductive reasoning. The patient must determine the need for additional information based on an analysis of the pertinent details. *The Syllogisms: If-Then Statements Series* provides useful stimuli for these tasks.

3.   The mediation of an argument requiring analysis and synthesis of information. Two points of view in a specific argument are presented. Using deductive reasoning, the premises or assumptions of each person must be considered in order to arrive at a solution. Once this is accomplished, the solution must be tested by analyzing the truth of the premises. Finally, utilizing complementary reasoning, a compromise must be negotiated based on the premises that are accepted and agreed to by both parties.

SELF-RELIANT FUNCTIONING (CARRY-OVER)

The final phase of our treatment addresses the carry-over of clinical tasks to functional, real-life situations. Our ultimate goal of therapy is to achieve maximum independence based on each patient's potential. When possible, patients are required to follow a schedule, maintain clothing and personal articles, request medication, handle money, prepare a daily log of activities, use the telephone, and identify emergency instructions. *The Amazing Adventures of Harvey Crumbaker: Skills for Living* addresses communication skills necessary for the foregoing situations. Home and community visits are important to test, refine, and adapt functional skills. Denial of deficits is often lessened as the patient encounters real-life situations.

Group therapy, in addition to individual therapy, is particularly important during this stage of treatment. Group therapy provides an opportunity for practice of learned skills, including the organization and articulation of thoughts, with individuals who are experiencing similar difficulties. Groups create a natural environment for interpersonal communication. Conversational skills include turn-taking, evaluating the speaker's intent, utilizing information appropriate to the knowledge and ability levels of listeners, self-monitoring, and the use and comprehension of gestures and intonational patterns. Through group feedback, peer pressure, and observations of other group members, the group, rather than the clinician, accepts the responsibility for increasing insight as well as the provision of rewards and support.

SELECTED REFERENCES

Baker, M. *Syllogisms: If-Then Statements.* Pacific Grove, California: Midwest Publications, 1981.

Folkes, J. *The Folkes Sentence Builder.* Hingham, Massachusetts: Teaching Resources Corp., 1981.

Hernadek, A. *Mind Benders: Deductive Thinking Skills.* Pacific Grove, California: Midwest Publications, 1978.

Klasky, C. *The Amazing Adventures of Harvey Crumbaker: Skills for Living.* Carson, California: Lakeshore Curriculum Materials Co., 1980.

Malkmus, D., Booth, D., and Kodimer, C. *Rehabilitation of the Head Injured Adult: Comprehensive Cognitive Management.* Downey, California: Rancho Los Amigos Hospital, Inc., 1980.

Ross, J., and Ross, C. *Ross Test of Higher Cognitive Processes.* New York: Slossen Educational Publications, Inc., 1976.

CHAPTER TWELVE

TREATMENT OF COMMUNICATION DISORDERS ASSOCIATED WITH GENERALIZED INTELLECTUAL DEFICITS IN ADULTS

Method of Lee Ann C. Golper and Marie T. Rau

The issue of "what to do" in the management of communication disorders occurring in association with generalized intellectual deficits, or secondary to a dementing disease, has become a topic of some debate among speech-language clinicians. It is generally agreed that when people have a moderate to severe memory impairment along with other cognitive deficits and, as is often the case with dementing illnesses, suffer from a progressive neurologic disease, their communication problems (1) are not the primary concern for patient care, and (2) are not likely to be changed by symptomatic therapies requiring adaptive learning. Nothing we have observed from working with patients who have generalized intellectual deficits, their families, or nursing staff personnel would cause us to feel that persons diagnosed as "demented" are particularly good candidates for learning adaptive or compensatory strategies to aid their communication. That is not to say, however, that a recommendation of "succor and comfort" should be the extent of appropriate treatment approaches for patients with generalized cognitive deficits. Having participated in geriatric teams and neurology consultation teams, we appreciate how specialists in communication disorders can substantially contribute to both the differential assessment and focus of therapies for intellectually impaired persons and their families.

THE DIAGNOSIS OF DEMENTIA

Table 1 serves to illustrate the range of disorders that can impair mental status. Persons who demonstrate an impairment in general intellectual abilities, or have the diagnosis of dementia, represent a vastly heterogeneous population. These individuals have in common

119

TABLE 1   Characteristics of Dementing Illnesses

Etiology of Dementia	*Primary Characteristics*
Multifocal Disorders (lacunar infarct syndrome, multiple, bilateral embolic and thrombo-embolic CVAs, vertebrobasilar disease, systemic lupus erythematosus, syphilis, anoxia)	"Patchy" neurologic deficits with some sensory, motor, or cognitive processes impaired and others spared Aphasia, dysarthria, or apraxia of speech may be present Impaired memory, attention, and learning abilities Onset of symptoms is abrupt and a step-wise deterioration will occur unless the disease process is controlled by medical management Most individuals are oriented and not confused, but they may lack awareness of their deficits
Diffuse pathologic states (metabolic disorders, postconcussive syndrome, normal pressure hydrocephalus, vitamin deficiencies, toxic conditions, infectious diseases, viral or bacterial encephalitis)	Acutely ill patients are often confused and disoriented Impaired memory and learning abilities Verbalizations and responses to questions will reflect a state of confusion and the patient's generally depressed mental status Onset of symptoms can be relatively abrupt, and there may be spontaneous recovery or remission of symptoms with medical therapies
Progressive subcortical dementias (Parkinson's disease, Huntington's disease, Wilson's disease, Creutzfeldt-Jacob's disease, progressive supranuclear palsy, subcortical gliosis, sarcoidosis, Wernicke's syndrome, Binswanger's disease)	Focal or generalized movement disorders can occur Progressively impaired memory and learning abilities with slowed thinking Dysarthrias are usually present Disturbances in emotional affect may be found Depending upon the illness, time of onset and rate of mental decline will vary
"Pseudodementia" depression or mood disorders (particularly in the elderly)	Motor speech and language abilities are unimpaired Complaints of memory impairment Patient displays signs of distress and has depressed affect Impairment is evident on memory and problem-tasks, but performance may improve with encouragement Cognitive abilities improve with medical management (antidepressant drugs) or psychological therapies for depression

TABLE 1   Characteristics of Dementing Illnesses (continued)

Etiology of Dementia	Primary Characteristics

Progressive degenerative dementia: Alzheimer's type (Alzheimer's disease, Pick's disease, senile dementia-Alzheimer's type)	Early characteristics
	  Personality changes and memory complaints
	  Impaired concentration
	  Reduced interest in family, vocation, and social achievement
	  Impaired memory and learning ability
	  Mild word-retrieval impairment
	  Difficulties with visuo-spatial tasks and abstract problem-solving
	Later characteristics
	  Disorientation and confusion
	  Global impairment in memory functions
	  Perseverative behavior
	  Motor unrest or lack of motor initiation
	  Relatively intact phonological or syntactic abilities with progressively impaired semantic abilities
	  Lack of ability to learn new skills or information
	End-stage characteristics
	  Inability to walk
	  Lack of sphincter control
	  "Aphasic-like" neologisms or jargon
	  Dysarthria
	  Lack of awareness of surroundings, others, and self

some degree of impaired memory, attention, and problem-solving ability. They have difficulty learning new information or acquiring new skills. These cognitive disorders are usually associated with decreased ability to independently manage functional activities of daily living. These behavioral disorders are usually the manifestation of diffuse neurologic diseases. In some cases the disturbances are the result of static or remitting conditions; however, the diagnosis of dementia is usually reserved for persons who have progressive, degenerative neurologic illnesses.

As Table 1 would suggest, the directions one might take in the management of a communication disorder associated with generalized intellectual impairment will vary, depending on (1) the etiology of the intellectual impairment and the subsequent prognosis for further mental declines, (2) the degree to which memory impairments affect adapative ability, (3) the degree to which attention and orientation are impaired, (4) the degree to which an individual demonstrates awareness or concern for his or her cognitive impairments, (5) the existence of any comcomitant sensory or motor deficit, (6) the counseling needs of the family, and (7) the degree to which the patient demonstrates a predominant speech or language disorder. It is obvious, therefore, that a determination of "what to do" in the management of intellectually impaired adults begins with a broad-based assessment protocol. We have found that a multi-disciplinary assessment procedure is the most efficient means for defining the problem areas, predicting outcomes, and outlining management plans.

Table 2 summarizes some of the information-gathering process. Like most medical facilities, we use a problem-oriented procedure

TABLE 2   Defining the Problems, Prognoses, and Treatment Plans

Neurologists, Psychiatrists or other physicians should:
  Provide a diagnosis of etiology
  Summarize the medical history
  Describe current medications and their effects on mentation and behavior
  Describe expected outcomes for medical therapies or the prognosis for remission or stabilization
    of symptoms
  Provide an assessment of mental status, sensory and motor functions

Psychologists should:
  Characterize the patient's memory impairments and other cognitive disorders
  Describe the patient's potential for adaptive learning
  Identify disturbances in mood or affective behavior
  Evaluate, conduct, or make recommendations for family counseling
  Direct behavioral intervention strategies in the home or nursing care facility

Speech-language pathologists should:
  Assess the nature of the patient's speech, language, functional and interpersonal communicative
    abilities
  Provide a differential diagnosis of the communication disorder
  Evaluate the patient's potential for learning adaptive communication strategies
  Provide treatment services or make recommendations to improve functional and interpersonal
    communicative abilities whenever practicable

Nursing care personnel, physical and occupational therapists should:
  Assess the patient's general functional abilities, including self care, transportation, bowel
    and bladder control, and social skills
  Identify fluctuations, if any, in the patient's behavior throughout the day
  Evaluate the degree of motor or sensory impairment and the potential for improved functioning
    with rehabilitation therapies
  Provide rehabilitation therapies or make any recommendations that might improve functional
    performance

Family members should:
  Describe the environmental and interpersonal situations within the home
  Discuss their interpretations and reactions to the patient's behavior
  Describe the history of the disorder
  Discuss their plans and placement alternatives they feel are appropriate to their needs and
    the needs of their impaired family member
  Discuss the degree to which they can observe or participate in recommended therapies
  Discuss their expectations for the patient

in which the primary diagnosis (e.g., multi-infarct dementia) is identified, and a list of patient, family, and staff problems is generated. Intervention objectives are then identified. It is important that these objectives be achievable therapeutic procedures, and not merely palliative recommendations.

What are some of the achievable therapeutic recommendations that can be made for communication disorders occurring in *association with,* or *secondary to,* generalized intellectual deficits? Whenever patients have obvious aphasic or dysarthric disorders complicated by disorders in attention, memory, and orientation, a revision or reassessment of therapy procedures is mandated. Any therapeutic approach that requires the learning of new behavior or purports to "stimulate" or re-establish previously learned abilities will, in large measure, be undermined by diffuse disease. Treatment, therefore, is better directed toward therapies that require little cognitive flexibility or learning. The therapies most likely to be recommended are highly pragmatic, that is, they are directed toward adjustments in the environment that can enhance functional and interpersonal communication, and ameliorate some of the concerns of the family or custodial personnel. A pragmatic approach to patient management has several advantages over more task-oriented or direct intervention strategies.

As was suggested at the outset, *talking* is not (or should not be) the major concern for patient management. When we receive a consult referral that states, "Aphasia secondary to organic brain syndrome—please evaluate for therapy," we can only assume the referring physician is having some difficulty communicating with the patient. Communication may be a relatively minor problem and "aphasia" may or may not be a part of the symptom complex. Patients' inability to comprehend and express themselves is, more often than not, a reflection of impaired memory, attention, and recognition of non-verbal as well as verbal stimuli. If they have a specific speech or language disorder overlaid upon other cognitive deficits, treatment should be approached cautiously. Practical management suggestions to improve functional communication may be warranted, and should be explored.

DIAGNOSTIC/PROGNOSTIC THERAPY

Patients whose generalized intellectual deficits are due to neurologic disorders that are static or remitting conditions, such as multiple infarctions or anoxic events, can be expected to demonstrate some degree of recovery. If speech or language abilities appear to be disproportionately depressed, relative to other functional abilities, an individual is seen for a brief period of diagnostic/prognostic treatment. The objectives of this treatment are (1) to characterize the essential features of the speech or language impairment and assess the influence of other cognitive deficits on communication, and (2) to examine the patient's ability to make use of intervention approaches to aid his or her speech intelligibiity, verbal formulation, or comprehension.

We have the advantagé of being able to conduct diagnostic/ prognostic therapy while the individuals are inpatients on a rehabilitation service or neurology ward. We can usually establish a prognosis for change with two to four weeks of daily patient visits. Although the majority of these patients are not recommended for a more extensive treatment regimen, spending time talking to them, cueing, or teaching specific tasks gives an opportunity to identify strategies that the families or custodial care personnel can use to best communicate with the impaired individual. If we find that the patients can communicate better with cues, such as redirecting them back to the topic, or using contextual cues to aid comprehension, we encourage the families or staff to observe the treatment session and use these strategies to talk to the patients. Just as with any other communicatively impaired population, we attempt to make the goals for this treatment service clear to the families and staff.

We explain that we will be making an appraisal of the problems and attempting to find the best way to communicate with the patient. We describe how our test results, the daily treatment data, and the evaluations and observations of other staff members will help us to determine whether or not speech-language therapies can make a difference in communicative abilities. It is our hope that diagnostic/ prognostic therapies will allow us to assess a patient's candidacy for further treatment services without encouraging unrealistic expectations for recovery. We would not initiate even the briefest period of diagnostic/prognostic therapy until patients appear to be "neurologically stable," that is, they have essentially recovered from the physiologic effects of an acute illness. Any amount of extended diagnostic or therapy services involves an investment of the resources, energy, and time of the patient, the family, and the clinician. The financial and other costs need to be carefully weighed against the anticipated outcome.

PROSTHETIC AIDS AND COMMUNICATION DEVICES

On occasion, the staff or family can be given certain practical therapeutic recommendations that will aid a patient's functional communication and do not require the learning of a new skill. It is amazing how often a speech-language pathologist is the first to suggest that some patients talk better, understand others, and orient to their surroundings better when they are sitting up, have properly functioning hearing aids, and are wearing their glasses and dentures. We recently evaluated an 82-year-old gentleman who had been in a motor vehicle accident. He was described as having "aphasia and dementia secondary to a postconcussive syndrome." After talking to the patient for a few minutes, we discovered that he had lost his glasses and hearing aid during the transfer from intensive care to the geriatric ward, and he had left his dentures at home. This patient had come to the United States from Sweden at age 19. His speech was mildly dysarthric and he had a pronounced Swedish accent. After he was fitted with a new hearing aid and glasses, his dentures were located, and we explained to the staff that he had a mild dysarthria and a Swedish accent, his "aphasia" resolved and his "dementia" dramatically improved.

This example points to the importance of inquiring about, or becoming sensitive to, symptoms which suggest that the patient has a visual or other sensory impairment. There have been patients who have come to our service wearing a malfunctioning hearing aid, usually due to a dead battery or clogged ear mold. If an individual is having difficulty driving a car or preparing a meal, one can reasonably assume that he or she might have some difficulty in properly cleaning and servicing a hearing aid, and that a family member or member of the nursing staff will need to assume the responsibility for its maintenance.

Aside from some of these obvious, but often overlooked, recommendations, we occasionally use prosthetic aids or nonverbal communication devices for patients who have motor speech disorders as a result of diffuse neurologic damage or a progressive neurologic disease. Candidates for these devices must be carefully selected. A palatal lift, for example, can often make a significant improvement in speech intelligibility for some types of dysarthria, but patients with generalized cognitive deficits may not tolerate the device, or fail to cooperate in using it consistently. Patients who suffer from progressive diseases often have, or later acquire, other oral movement deficits so that devices for velopharyngeal closure may not dramatically improve intelligibility.

Our experience has demonstrated that there is a great deal of variation in the course of some of the progressive subcortical dementias, both across etiologies and among individuals. In some cases the patient's general mental status is not dramatically impaired until the end stages of the disease. The patient may have impairments in swallowing or speech intelligibility that are a primary concern for management. In our facility we use cinefluorographic studies to evaluate swallowing behavior and to make recommendations for food placement, type of diet, and posture or swallowing therapies that will reduce the possibility of aspiration. If patients are unable to convey their wants to the nursing staff, we usualy provide them with some type of nonvocal communication device. The devices are selected depending on the individual's manual dexterity, degree of residual intelligible speech, and ability to learn a new skill. Usually spelling boards are provided to augment the speech attempts of patients with moderately decreased intelligibility. More severely impaired persons are given devices that utilize picture displays, since they require fewer movements to convey a message. A few sessions of bedside therapy, with the family and staff in attendance, helps us to determine whether the patient can make use of the device.

As stated earlier, we can sometimes produce an improvement in the patient's functional communication with some very practical observations and recommendations. Although these recommendations may be patently obvious to a specialist in communication disorders, they may not have been considered by the family or other staff members. When an individual has a chronic, severe intellectual deficit, or a progressive disease, the suggestions speech-language pathologists make—and the prostheses or communication aids we supply—may not have a significant or lasting effect on functional communication. Still, if we feel a patient might benefit from the use of a relatively inexpensive communication aid, even for a few weeks or months, we would certainly recommend its use.

ENVIRONMENTAL ADJUSTMENTS AND STIMULATION THERAPIES

The neurologic disease we most often associate with dementia is Alzheimer's disease, or Alzheimer's-type senile dementia. This disorder is insidious in its onset, with memory loss and personality changes, being the earliest complaints. As the disease progresses, patients may complain about, or demonstrate, word-retrieval deficits. In the later stages, verbal perseverations, stereotypic utterances, and "aphasic-like" neologisms may be found. Although language abilities, particularly semantic abilities, will inevitably be eroded by this progressive disease, we cannot imagine an instance in which specific speech-language therapies would be recommended.

Depending on the patient's living situation and the degree of dementia, there may be some environmental adjustments recommended that will help the impaired individual maintain functional living activities as long as possible. The sorts of suggestions that have been offered by the psychologist and others stress the importance of allowing the patients to do as much for themselves as possible, and of maintaining a structured routine in the home or nursing care facility. Families and nursing care staff are advised to encourage patients to complete tasks, such as dressing themselves, even though it may require giving short, simple "one-step-at-a-time" directions. We advise keeping clocks and calendars within the room, and signs or pictures on bathroom and closet doors, to keep the patient oriented. We explain to families that transferring a patient from the home environment to a hospital or nursing home will usually precipitate a marked decline in functional abilities and orientation, at least temporarily.

The psychologist recommends maintaining a stimulating, non-fatiguing environment. Conversations with the patient are an excellent stimulation therapy. We advise families to talk to their impaired family member about activities in the hospital or nursing home. We suggest that they talk about activities the patient has continued to enjoy, such as watching television, looking at magazines, listening to music, and so forth. Looking through an album of family photographs can be a productive conversational stimulation activity. The purpose of these recommendations is twofold. First, they give the family directions to follow at a time when they feel guilty if they are not "doing something" to help their impaired family member. Second, they give the patient the advantage of some degree of independence (however marginal) and opportunities for conversational interactions.

SPOUSE/FAMILY COUNSELING THERAPIES

Our facility conducts a weekly spouse/family counseling group staffed by two neuropsychologists and a speech-language pathologist. This group is directed toward the educational and counseling needs of the spouses and family members of persons who have chronic neurologic diseases. It is our feeling that we can often do a great deal more for the families than for the patients themselves. This group affords families an opportunity to discuss their concerns, experiences, and feelings. Families can interact with others who share similar problems, and this discussion provides a measure of support for those who are coping with the crisis of nursing home placement or "role reversals" within the home. The clinicians discuss the causes for changes in behavior, such as emotional lability or changes in sexual activities. They provide an avenue for families to ask questions about a particular disease and give them the information and support they need to make whatever homelife adjustments may be necessary. Communication is an important activity for families as well as patients. We strongly encourage families to participate in our spouse/family counseling group, or we refer them to other support groups, self-help groups, and professionals in the community.

SUMMARY

We have briefly described here some of what our service does, in concert with other professional staff and families, when an individual has a communication disorder associated with generalized cognitive deficits. We do not attempt to place patients in a treatment program for which they lack the requisite skills to succeed. Aphasia therapies are designed for aphasic persons; that is, persons who have the residual abilities to acquire alternative strategies to communicate. We work in a setting that extends clinical services to older populations and to adults with a variety of neurologic diseases. "Purely" dysarthric or aphasic conditions are a minority of our diagnostic and treatment referrals. This is due, perhaps, to the active participation of our service in geriatric and neurology teams providing services to the communicatively handicapped geriatric patient. Since neurologic diseases are seldom polite enough to impair only language or speech functions (and epidemiologic evidence suggests that a good percentage of persons over 65 will have clinically important intellectual deficits), we suspect that most clinicians in hospitals, rehabilitation programs, or nursing home facilities face many of the same diagnostic enigmas and treatment challenges we face when providing services to the geriatric patient.

In determining the options for therapy for intellectually impaired patients, we look first at the boundaries and then at the horizons. We ask, "Does this patient have a predominant speech or language disorder that is discrepant with his or her other cognitive or functional living abilities? What is the predicted outcome for the underlying neurologic disease? Are there any practical recommendations or environmental adjustments that can be made to aid this patient's functional communication?'' Finally, we ask, ''What are the educational and counseling needs of the family?''

We see the role of speech-language pathologists in the management of persons with generalized intellectual deficits as primarily a diagnostic and prognostic service, but we can play an equally important role as a consultant to the staff and families. Our facility places a high value on the importance of communication between and among the staff, the patient, and the family. Our treatment options are not ''language'' or ''speech'' therapies; they are *conjoint counseling* and *communication therapies* for the patients and all those concerned with their care.

SELECTED REFERENCES

Eisdorfer, C., and Stotsky, B. Intervention treatment and rehabilitation of psychiatric disorders. In J. Birren and K. Schaie (Eds.). *Handbook of the Psychology of Aging.* New York: Van Nostrand Reinhold Company, 1977.

Golper, L., and Binder, L. Communicative behavior in aging and dementia. In J. Darby (Ed.), *Speech Assessment in Medicine and Psychiatry.* Volume 2. New York: Grune and Stratton, 1981.

Johns, D. (Ed.), *Clinical Management of Neurogenic Communicative Disorders.* Boston: Little, Brown and Company, 1978.

National Institute of Aging Task Force. Senility reconsidered: Treatment possibilities for mental impairment in the elderly. *Journal of the American Medical Association,* 1980, *244,* 259–263.

Slaby, A., and Wyatt, R. *Dementia in the Presenium.* Springfield, Illinois: Charles C. Thomas, 1974.

CHAPTER THIRTEEN

TREATMENT OF DIALECTAL DIFFERENCES OF SOCIOLINGUISTIC ORIGIN

Method of Joan C. Payne-Johnson

During my professional tenure, a number of speech/language pathologists have expressed their concern to me about the appropriateness of therapy for persons who have been diagnosed as having culturally different dialects. The nature of the problem, as it has been expressed, is that there is no sharp line of demarcation between the responsibilities of the reading teacher, the teacher of English, the teacher of speech or language arts, and the speech/language pathologist as to who should assist culturally different persons, whose first language is English, to develop expertise in Standard English.

Another facet of the dilemma here is that a great deal of controversial discussion was under way during the renaissance of the sixties about the nature of the culturally different dialect of black Americans and the approaches one should take for therapeutic intervention. The relevancy of educational strategies for dialectal differences was subject to much debate in terms of the need to teach speakers to "code-switch" dialect and Standard English, according to the context of the situation.

The issue was then, and still is, a highly charged sociopolitical matter with strong overtones of listener bias against those who represent culturally or ethnically different communities. The irony is that, with all of the scholarly philosophizing on the history, causes, and features of culturally different dialects, persons who should be in the process of, or who are actively engaged in, becoming speakers of Standard English, in addition to their dialect, are perhaps not getting the kind of specialized help from teachers or clinicians to make the transition.

Perhaps part of the hesitancy of speech/language pathologists to include dialectal differences of sociolinguistic origin in their caseloads is that ours is a profession that treats handicaps in communication. Consequently, when we apply a pathological connotation to the word "handicap," a dialectal difference would obviously disqualify an individual from receiving services from specialists in our discipline. On the other hand, if we conceptualize "handicap" as including those psychological or economic penalties imposed upon a speaker because he or she is different from the norm, in this case Standard English speakers, then we have broadened our charge and our responsibilities. Assuming that all persons aspire to the highest quality of life that hard work, talents, and abilities can provide, then any obstacle to those aspirations, because of a difference in style of speech, may be considered a handicapping condition and is within the purview of our profession.

The nature of my clinical experiences in the inner city and on the campus of a historically black institution prompts me to say, foremost, that the effectiveness of any program of intervention lies in the cultural sensitivity of the clinician. As in any other form of verbal expression, dialectal variation is systematic, rule-governed, and deeply embedded in the cultural experiences of the speaker. Moreover, dialectal variations are positively reinforced in the community in which the speaker lives; the dialectal system emanates from a community of people who share, with the speaker, a common frame of reference. To denigrate in any way the existing dialect, is to speak pejoratively of the speaker and of all that has value for him. My experience has shown that the clinician must understand these factors if analysis of the dialect and intervention are to be efficacious.

Inasmuch as we are not treating a pathological condition, we are not called upon to devote hours of intensive therapy to enable the client to communicate. Effective informal communication to a fairly large number of persons has already been established; it is another level of communication we wish to add to the speaker's linguistic repertoire. It should be considered that the percentage of dialectal variation, when compared to the total discourse of the speaker, will be relatively small. In the case of the black dialect speaker (and not all black speakers are speakers of a different dialect), current research has identified those parameters of dialect that appear with regularity. These differences are in the copula verb "to be," in subject-verb agreement, in verb tense, in the use of possessive markers, and in sound substitutions.

In the main, however, the conversational speech is the same as that of the Standard English speaker. There may also be some non-verbal differences in inflection, for example, which may alter the meanings of words, and there may be some differences in thinking that are firmly entrenched in regional and cultural experiences unique to some communities. I advise the clinician to distinguish between the systematic dialectal variations and any paralinguistic or transient elements of speech (slang, for example), which are part of the client's group identification.

In pointing out that there are some differences between the culturally different dialect of many black speakers and speakers of Standard English, one can make a case for counseling and self-management as positive strategies. These procedures are applicable to all culturally different dialects, and a similar therapeutic model has already been described (Seymour and Seymour, 1977). The approach is to:

1.   Listen to and isolate those features that appear with regularity in the dialect. Separate these from the slang and idiomatic expressions that are transient and unique to the region or to a subculture of the community.

2.   Listen to the speaker and, in the case of an unfamiliar dialect, to the speaking patterns of family members. As with #1, listen and isolate dialectal differences from other elements of speech.

3.   Compare the dialectal features with their counterparts in Standard English.

4.   Develop visual and auditory aids that demonstrate the parallels between dialectal features and their Standard English counterparts.

5.   Counsel the client on the settings in which the cultural dialect, or informal pattern, is acceptable, and contrast these with those settings in which Standard English, the formal pattern of speech, is expected.

6.   Provide the client with opportunities to practice, using Standard English exclusively.

7.   Role-play situations in which the culturally different dialect may be used. Have the client practice speaking in those situations.

8.   Encourage the client to develop his or her own checklist or guide for self-monitoring in carry-over situations.

9.   Arrange for periodic progress reports and re-evaluations once the client has demonstrated proficiency in using both the dialect and Standard English in the prescribed settings.

I stress the sharing of the therapy experience with the client's family and significant others, where possible, with the full understanding that those closest to the client may be very resistant to any efforts to change the familiar speech. It has been my experience that when the culturally different dialect speaker goes back to the community in which everyone else speaks the dialect, carry-over may be negligible in the face of family or peer-group pressure to maintain the interpersonal status quo. I would suggest, however, that it is in the client's best interests for the clinician to work on sharing the goals of therapy with those persons who have a significant relationship to the speaker. Whenever possible, the family should be made aware that the effort is to teach the client—without eliminating the familiar dialect—to fit linguistic codes to specific settings. During family counseling, the benefits to the client's education or employment should be highlighted, inasmuch as this kind of therapeutic intervention may also translate into better grades or greater upward mobility.

Finally, I would strongly urge that, for school-aged clients, the speech/language pathologist establish and maintain cooperative management arrangements with the reading teacher and the teacher of English. Dialectal differences are manifested in reading and writing, as well as in speech, and it will be useful to share progress in therapy with the other professionals who are working with the client's ability to use Standard English.

This program of intervention underscores the clinician's sensitivity to cultures and life-styles that may be at variance with her or his own. This is not necessarily an approach advocated by the many who feel that any form of intervention tampers with the individual's cultural integrity. However, it represents a compromise on behalf of the client to enable him to make choices and decisions based on the knowledge of linguistic flexibility.

SELECTED REFERENCES

Seymour, H. and Seymour, C. A therapeutic model for communication disorders among children who speak Black English vernacular. *Journal of Speech and Hearing Disorders,* 1977, *42:* 238–246.

Smitherman, G. *Talking and Testifying: The Language of Black America.* Boston: Houghton Mifflin, 1977.

CHAPTER 12

CHAPTER FOURTEEN

EVALUATION OF TREATMENT OF ADULTS WITH LANGUAGE DISORDERS

Method of Kathryn M. Yorkston

Although the focus of this chapter will be on the measures of treatment effectiveness in the clinical setting, I will begin by discussing a general approach to the study of treatment efficacy. Traditionally, the question has been posed in the following way, "Is treatment effective for the average aphasic patient?" Answering this general question requires that carefully selected groups of treated and untreated patients be tested, by means of standardized procedures, throughout the course of recovery. Results are compared to determine differences in recovery between the groups. Although a large-scale efficacy study is currently being undertaken in the VA Cooperative project, such well-controlled studies are difficult to carry out. Care is needed to control a number of variables that have the potential for effecting the outcome—including age, sex, education, etiology, time since onset, and site of lesion. Further, application of the results of group efficacy studies to the clinical setting is limited by the need to interpret the results in statistical terms. For example, the trend toward improved performance with treatment for the average patient does not allow the clinician to make definitive statements about the effect of treatment on the individual patient. Also, statistically significant group performance differences may or may not be clinically important. It is possible for a small improvement in scores—consistent across subjects—to be statistically significant but functionally unimportant.

Although the usefulness of the general approach to efficacy studies cannot be overlooked, clearly this approach is not sufficient for clinical purposes. The general approach must be supplemented by other techniques to answer certain critical clinical questions. I use a variety of measurement techniques, which combine to serve at least three purposes: (1) to indicate changes in an aphasic individual's performance, (2) to assess the impact of treatment upon that change, and (3) to measure the impact of changing performance on functional communication skills.

STANDARDIZED APHASIA BATTERIES

A number of standardized test batteries are available. Among them are the Boston Diagnostic Aphasia Examination (BDAE), the Minnesota Test for Differential Diagnosis of Aphasia, and the Porch Index of Communicative Abilities (PICA). These batteries consist of a number of language-related tasks sampling speaking, listening, reading, and writing skills. Tasks vary from simple (matching identical objects) to difficult (verbally retelling a story which has been read). Performance is scored in a plus/minus fashion, on a rating scale, or on a multidimensional scoring system, which takes into account completeness, promptness, and responsiveness, as well as accuracy. Of course, it is beyond the scope of this chapter to review existing aphasia batteries; that has been done elsewhere (Linebaugh, 1979). Rather, it is the purpose of this discussion to describe how standardized tests can be used in the clinical setting.

During the initial evaluation, I make the selection of the standardized test, depending upon the specific questions being asked. For example, the BDAE is particularly useful in addressing issues of differential diagnosis such as: "Does this patient exhibit aphasia?" and "If so, how severe is the disorder, and what type of aphasia does it represent?" Any of the standard batteries that sample a large number of tasks at various difficulty levels may be used to ask such treatment-planning questions as: "Is treatment appropriate?" and "If so, what would be an appropriate treatment focus?" I find the PICA particularly useful as a measure of subtle changes in performance over time. When administered on a monthly basis, results of the PICA can be used to answer the question, "Are the language skills of this patient changing?"

Before discussing the specifics of how standardized test results can measure treatment effectiveness, I will review the general characteristics of these batteries, which allow them to serve this purpose. First, they sample many different language tasks representing a wide range of difficulty levels. This is necessary, since aphasia may cross all language modalities and vary from mild to severe. Ideally, a test battery administered to a patient would include tasks sampling different language skills at three difficulty levels: those difficult enough to produce consistent errors; those in which the patient makes some correct response, but exhibits processing problems such as delayed or corrected attempts; and those easy enough for the patients' responses to be essentially normal. Second, standardized test batteries prescribe administration and scoring procedures in order to ensure uniformity. Such uniformity is critical for reliability when comparisons are to be made across time. Finally, standardized tests are designed to be sensitive to small changes in performance. Different test batteries handle the issue of sensitivity in different ways. Some tests sample large numbers of tasks and items. Others achieve sensitivity by scoring many aspects of patients' behavior on a relatively small number of tasks.

I find several aspects of the results of standardized testing particularly useful as indicators of a patient's changing performance.

1. *Overall improvement.* Many test batteries result in a single overall score. For example, the results of the PICA are reported as a percentile score, comparing a patient's overall performance with a large number of left-hemisphere-damaged individuals. Improvement in overall scores gives a gross indication of magnitude of change.

2. *Pattern of improvement.* I look for improvement on specific tasks for two reasons. First, important changes on specific tasks may be "washed-out," if only overall scores are examined. Overall scores must reflect performance on all tasks, including those that are either so easy or so difficult that they are not sensitive to change. Second, I am interested in changing performance on tasks similar, but not identical, to those that have been the focus of treatment attention. For example, if auditory comprehension has been the focus of treatment during the interval since the last testing, I look for verification of treatment effectiveness to tasks that depend heavily on auditory comprehension skills, despite the fact that the tasks themselves may not be identical to the tasks actually used in treatment.

3. *Processing behaviors.* Communication performance of aphasic patients is often characterized by what may be called "overt processing behaviors." These behaviors reflect reduced ability to handle language tasks. They may include delayed or distorted responses, correction attempts when errors are recognized, ability to retrieve words only when supplied with semantic or phonemic cues, or requests for repetition of stimuli. I look for changes in a patient's processing behavior as an indicator of changing skills. I will illustrate this concept by discussing changes in processing behavior typically seen on a single task as recovery occurs. Initially, the task may be so difficult that no overt processing behaviors are apparent. In this case, the patient's performance may be similar on all items and may be characterized by rejection of the task or by consistent unrecognized errors. As recovery occurs and the task becomes less difficult, performance may become less consistent. For example, the patient may begin to correct some of the errors, may take much longer to respond, or may indicate in some way that an attempt is being made to cue

the correct response. As further recovery occurs, the processing behaviors again become less apparent. As a task becomes easy, the patient's overt behavior is no longer giving information about how the task is being processed. In some test batteries, for example, the PICA, quantification of processing behaviors is formally incorporated into the multidimensional scoring system. In other batteries, quantification of these behaviors is done informally. Careful examination of a patient's processing behavior across a variety of tasks not only indicates changing skills, but also leads to selection of appropriate treatment tasks.

In summary, standardized test batteries are useful in that they allow the clinician to sample a broad range of communication tasks, and to obtain reproducible results that give a reliable indication of overall level of performance, patterns of relative task difficulty, and changing communication skills. However, certain issues are not easily addressed through examination of the results of standardized test batteries. First, although batteries contain tasks that adequately sample the communication behavior of the majority of aphasic individuals, standardized testing may not be appropriate for groups of patients at either end of the severity continuum. The behaviors of severely involved patients who are unable to perform tasks included in formal batteries might be more productively analyzed in natural communication environments. On the other end of the continuum, mildly involved patients may perform normally on tasks included in standard batteries. Thus reading, listening, speaking, and writing tasks that are more taxing must be found to serve as monitors of change. Second, changes in performance on standardized tasks based on a stimulus-response model may or may not reflect changing performance in functional, interactive communication. Finally, although results of standardized batteries are useful as an indicator of whether or not change is occurring, the question, "Is this patient recovering?" is different from "Is treatment helping this patient to recover?" The relative contribution of spontaneous recovery and aphasia treatment to recovery is a traditionally troublesome one, and cannot easily be addressed through the standardized testing of individual patients in the clinical setting. The following discussion will deal more directly with techniques that assess the specific impact of treatment and distinguish it from the influence of other factors, including spontaneous recovery.

MONITORING CHANGE THROUGH TREATMENT TASKS

Measurement of performance on treatment tasks is a useful means of assessing effectiveness of that treatment. It is beyond the scope of this chapter to present a detailed analysis of task selection. However, since measurement of tasks leads directly from the types of tasks employed, it is necessary to briefly discuss some general principles of task selection. I select tasks with two questions in mind. First, is the aphasic patient able to actively process the task? Using this principle, tasks that are easy enough to allow the patient to respond accurately "without thinking" are eliminated. Likewise, tasks so difficult that the patient is unable to process them are eliminated. Second, does increased accuracy and efficiency in performing this task have a potential impact on the patient's ability to function in ordinary situations?

In order to illustrate different approaches to the measurement of performance on a single task, I will present a common treatment task similar to those described by Davis and Wilcox in PACE therapy. The aphasic patient draws a picture from a deck containing a series of pictures of common objects, and attempts to communicate to the clinician the name of the object. In order to simulate natural communication, the clinician remains naive to the specific word that the aphasic is trying to communicate and so does not look at the picture. If the aphasic speaker is not readily able to communicate the correct information, the clinician and aphasic speaker are free to interact in a question-and-answer format until the name of the object is communicated. Performance on this naming task can be measured in a number of ways:

1. *Accuracy*. Perhaps the simplest measure of performance on this task is the percentage of object names the aphasic speaker is able to communicate accurately. Increases in accuracy indicate improving performance. However, accuracy alone does not provide complete clinical information. If only those tasks with high levels of accuracy (80 to 90 percent) are selected in treatment, accuracy scores soon reach the ceiling level of 100 percent. If accuracy were the only measure being considered when making program change decisions, more difficult tasks probably would be selected after several consecutive days of accurate performance. In many instances this would be inappropriate. Although the patients may achieve ceiling accuracy scores, the performance may be deficient in terms of a number of other dimensions including rate, the need for clinician cueing, and self-corrected responses. Therefore, I find accuracy more

useful as a measure of task appropriateness (with high scores indicating that the patient is able to process the task) than as a measure of improvement.

2. *Processing Behaviors.* Quantification of the frequency of occurrence and type of processing behaviors that were described earlier is a useful indicator of changing performance. In order to quantify the naming task presented earlier, I would develop a simple coding system reflecting some frequently occurring processing behaviors. For example, each accurate response might be coded as "d" if it was delayed, as "c" if clinician cues were needed, and as "cr" if the patient corrected an initially erroneous response. Improvement on this task could be documented by identifying decreases in the number of processing behaviors, or by a shift in the type of processing behaviors moving away from clinician-dependent behavior to more independent retrieval strategies. Such coding systems are developed individually, depending on the patient and task.

3. *Efficiency.* The third measure of changing performance is the efficiency with which a patient is able to perform a specific task. Clinically, I define efficiency as the rate of accurate performance on a task. Efficiency can be computed by dividing the number of correct responses by the total time, in order to obtain a measure of accurate responses per minute. One of the benefits of supplementing the measure of accuracy with rate is that it allows the clinician to see changing performance, despite the patient's performance at near ceiling level for accuracy. In other words, a patient who is able to communicate 15 object names per minute clearly is performing better than one who is able to communicate only five names per minute, despite the fact that both may be 100 percent accurate in their responses. Further, efficiency reflects the processing behaviors by measuring the time required for a response, which increases depending on difficulty of retrieval. Measures of efficiency are relatively simple to obtain, can be computed in a few seconds, and apply to a wide variety of patients and tasks.

Turning away from *what* measures to obtain, I will now discuss the issue of how to use these measures to clinically address pertinent questions related to the effectiveness of treatment. Several useful techniques fall under the heading of clinical research or single-case research design.

1. *Serial measurement.* This technique involves obtaining repetitive performance measures during a period of treatment. Using as an example the task described earlier, a series of measures of

efficiency might be obtained daily on a ten-item probe. Increasing efficiency scores would indicate that the patient's skills on this task are changing. However, serial measures of performance do not allow you to ask the clinically critical question, "Are skills changing as a result of the treatment?"

2. *Baseline designs.* This technique involves a period of pretreatment monitoring of performance in which several measures of object naming might be obtained before initiation of a treatment program. I look at two types of information as a measure of effectiveness of treatment. The first is a comparison of the average level of performance during the baseline period with that of the treatment period. I use this as a general indicator of whether or not change is occurring, regardless of what is causing it. The second pertinent comparison is the rate at which the performance is changing during baseline, as opposed to the treatment period. Since we often work with patients whose performance is changing spontaneously, a more rapid rate of change during treatment would indicate that treatment is facilitating recovery.

3. *Withdrawal designs.* This technique involves alternating periods of treatment, called the "A" phase, and no treatment, called the "B" phase. So, "BABA" design would include a baseline, a treatment, a no-treatment, and a second treatment phase. One advantage of the withdrawal over the baseline design is the more rigorous confirmation of treatment effectiveness. However, clinically, an extended period of behavioral monitoring without treatment may be troublesome. Further, this technique is more easily interpreted when the treatment effect is reversible; that is, performance is expected to go back to baseline when treatment is removed. This is not the case with most aphasia treatment.

4. *Multiple baseline designs.* This technique involves the monitoring of baseline performance on several tasks, then staggering the initiation of treatment. In other words, baselines are continuing on task B and C while treatment is beginning on A, and later, baseline continues on task C as treatment is continuing on A and beginning on B. I will use the object-naming task to illustrate some possible applications of multiple baseline designs. If the question of generalization of learning is important, a large number of pictures might be divided into several similar groups. Baseline measures would initially be taken on all groups of pictures, then initiation of training on each group would begin in a staggered fashion. Performance levels on treated pictures could be compared to untreated pictures and to pretreatment baseline measure on treated pictures. If performance on untreated words increases faster than it did during

baseline, one assumes that some generalization of training from the treatment has occurred. If the question of relative effectiveness of two different cueing strategies is important, a multiple baseline technique could be used to compare rates of performance change between two treatment approaches.

Clearly, with single case designs, particular questions and tasks need to be individualized. Further goals need to be determined on a case-by-case basis. Rarely is it useful to apply statistical methods in single-case design; rather, target performance levels are set relative to clinically or functionally important measures.

MEASURES OF FUNCTIONAL COMMUNICATION

The last topic approaches the efficacy question from a slightly different perspective; that is, "Does treatment allow this patient to function better in ordinary situations?" No doubt this is the most difficult of the efficacy issues, but it is also the most fundamental. Increased performance on standardized test batteries or on treatment tasks is encouraging, but carries little meaning if it is not accompanied by improved performance in ordinary communicative situations. Measures of treatment effectiveness in natural settings can be obtained through standardized tests such as Holland's Communication Activities of Daily Living or Sarno's Functional Communication Profile. Also, natural communication activities can be simulated using treatment tasks like those suggested by Davis and Wilcox in PACE therapy.

I videotape standard interactions between clinician and aphasic patient, or between spouse and aphasic patient. One such type of interaction requires the communication partner to elicit information from the aphasic patient about a picture that the partner cannot see. The videotapes are reviewed to identify the strategies, used by the aphasic patient and the communication partner, that appear to either impede or facilitate the communication process. Review of the taped interactions serves as the basis for spouse counseling as well as documentation of the changing performance of the aphasic individual. Although functional communication tasks are receiving increased attention in research and clinical literature, natural communication interactions are difficult to objectively quantify. Any quantification system must reflect the complex interactive process, which requires that both partners listen and speak, take turns exchanging information, and confirm previously established information. Clearly, measures of natural communication are important. However, clinically applicable techniques for describing and precisely quantifying this type of communication await future research development.

SELECTED REFERENCES

Davis, G. and Wilcox, M. Incorporating parameters of natural conversation in aphasia treatment: PACE therapy. In R. Chapey (Ed.), *Language Intervention Strategies in Adult Aphasia*. Baltimore: Williams & Wilkins, 1981.

Hersen, M., and Barlow, D. *Single Case Experimental Designs: Strategies for Studying Behavior Change*. New York: Pergamon Press, 1976.

Linebaugh, C. Assessing the assessments: The adequacy of standardized tests of aphasia. In R. Brookshire (Ed.), *Clinical Aphasiology: Proceedings of the Conference 1979*. Minneapolis: BRK Publishers, 8–22, 1979.

Marshall, R., and Tomkins, C. Identifying behavior associated with verbal self-correction of aphasic clients. *Journal of Speech and Hearing Disorders*. 1981, 46:168–173.

Silverman, F. *Research Design in Speech Pathology and Audiology*. Englewood Cliffs, New Jersey: Prentice-Hall, Inc., 1977.

Acknowledgment: This study was supported in part by Research Grant #G008003029 from the National Institute of Handicapped Research, Department of Education, Washington, D.C. 20202.

INDEX